FUTURE ANESTHESIA DELIVERY SYSTEMS

FUTURE ANESTHESIA DELIVERY SYSTEMS

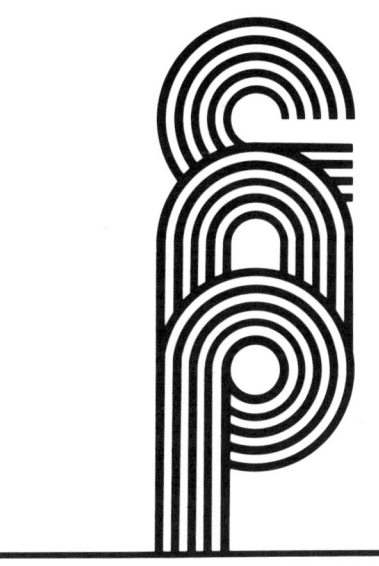

CONTEMPORARY

ANESTHESIA

PRACTICE

BURNELL R. BROWN, JR., EDITOR

JERRY M. CALKINS, Ph.D., M.D., and
REYNOLDS J. SAUNDERS, M.D.,
ASSOCIATE EDITORS

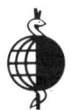 F. A. DAVIS COMPANY / PHILADELPHIA

Copyright © 1984 by F. A. Davis Company

All rights reserved. This book is protected by copyright. No part of it may be reproduced, stored in a retrieval system, or transmitted in any form or by any means, electronic, mechanical, photocopying, recording, or otherwise, without written permission from the publisher.

Printed in the United States of America

Library of Congress Cataloging in Publication Data
Main entry under title:

Future anesthesia delivery systems.

(Contemporary anesthesia practice ; v. 8)
Includes bibliographical references and index.
1. Anesthesiology—Apparatus and instruments. 2. Anesthesiology. I. Brown, Burnell R. II. Calkins, Jerry M. III. Saunders, Reynolds J. IV. Series. [DNLM: 1. Anesthesia—Methods. 2. Anesthesiology—Instrumentation. 3. Technology, Medical. 4. Anesthesia—Trends. W1 CO769ME v.8 / WO 240 F996]
RD78.8.F87 1984   617'.97   83-7844
ISBN 0-8036-1277-X

PREFACE

With recent advances in technology, an overwhelming number of new developments in anesthesia equipment are being introduced to the market. Many of these new developments have centered around patient monitoring and instrumentation. For a number of reasons that are quite complex, interrelated, and multifaceted, application of technology to the design of new anesthesia delivery systems (i.e., gas machines) has been lacking.

Numerous books have been written discussing monitoring and its wide applications to anesthesia. While a few books have discussed in significant detail the features and construction of current anesthesia equipment, little has been written or summarized regarding future design concepts of anesthesia delivery systems.

This book articulates principles of anesthesia system design and provides examples of their implementation in delivery systems devised by noted investigators in anesthesia delivery. To accomplish this, four major topic areas have been addressed. The first section deals with problems and controversies in anesthetic delivery. Here the needs for new systems, for computers, for standards, and for alternatives of closed and semiclosed anesthesia delivery are discussed. Presentation of these controversies sets the stage for the next section, which explores what we know about the designs of the future and what functions the various subsystems or components of any future anesthetic machine design are going to have to accomplish. These functions include anesthetic gas and vapor delivery, waste gas recovery, control of anesthesia delivery, monitoring of system gas concentrations, ventilation of the patient, and automation and computerization of data gathering, analysis, and record-keeping. The third section presents designs of prototypes by selected groups who have been involved with the development of anesthesia delivery systems. These include the Boston Anesthesia System, the Arizona System, the Alabama System, and the Utah System. The last section deals with what we as anesthesiologists can do until the future arrives. How do we assess equipment? And how do we decide what is necessary?

Jerry M. Calkins, Ph.D., M.D.
Reynolds J. Saunders, M.D.

CONTRIBUTORS

Walter J. Arnell, Ph.D.
Professor of Systems and Industrial Engineering
College of Engineering
University of Arizona
Tucson, AZ

Burnell R. Brown, Jr., M.D., Ph.D.
Professor and Chairman
Department of Anesthesiology
University of Arizona Health Sciences Center
Tucson, AZ

Jerry M. Calkins, Ph.D., M.D.
Assistant Professor
Department of Anesthesiology
University of Arizona Health Sciences Center
Tucson, AZ

Jeffrey B. Cooper, Ph.D.
Associate Director
Department of Biomedical Engineering
Massachusetts General Hospital
Assistant Professor of Anesthesia
Harvard Medical School
Boston, MA

Edward A. Ernst, M.D.
Professor and Chairman
Department of Anesthesiology
University of Alabama School of Medicine
Birmingham, AL

Thomas C. Jannett, M.S.
Associate Professor
Department of Anesthesiology
University of Alabama School of Medicine
Birmingham, AL

Warren R. Jewett, Sc.D.
Department of Electrical Engineering
University of Arizona
Tucson, AZ

William S. Jordan, M.D.
Associate Professor
Department of Anesthesiology
University of Utah College of Medicine
Salt Lake City, UT

Kenneth C. Mylrea, Ph.D.
Associate Professor
Department of Electrical Engineering
College of Engineering
University of Arizona
Tucson, AZ

Ronald S. Newbower, Ph.D.
Acting Director
Department of Biomedical Engineering
Massachusetts General Hospital
Assistant Professor of Anesthesia
Harvard Medical School
Boston, MA

Charles W. Otto, M.D.
Associate Professor
Department of Anesthesiology
University of Arizona Health Sciences Center
Tucson, AZ

Leslie Rendell-Baker, M.D.
Professor of Anesthesiology
Loma Linda University School of Medicine
Loma Linda VA Hospital
Loma Linda, CA

Reynolds J. Saunders, M.D.
Lecturer
Department of Anesthesiology
University of Arizona Health Sciences Center
Chief, Anesthesia Service
VA Hospital
Tucson, AZ

Donald G. Schultz, Ph.D.
Professor
Department of Systems and Industrial Engineering
College of Engineering
University of Arizona
Tucson, AZ

Jeffry A. Spain, M.D.
Instructor
Department of Anesthesiology
University of Arizona Health Sciences Center
Tucson, AZ

Charles K. Waterson, B.S.E.
Research Assistant
Department of Anesthesiology
University of Arizona Health Sciences Center
Tucson, AZ

Dwayne R. Westenskow, Ph.D.
Associate Professor
Department of Anesthesiology
University of Utah College of Medicine
Salt Lake City, UT

CONTENTS

SECTION 1. PROBLEMS AND CONTROVERSIES IN ANESTHETIC DELIVERY   1

    1. WHY NEW DELIVERY SYSTEMS?   3
   Jerry M. Calkins, Ph.D., M.D.

    2. CLOSED-CIRCUIT AND HIGH-FLOW SYSTEMS: EXAMINING ALTERNATIVES   11
   Edward A. Ernst, M.D., and Jeffry A. Spain, M.D.

    3. COMPUTERS: DO WE NEED THEM NOW?   39
   Jeffry A. Spain, M.D., and Reynolds J. Saunders, M.D.

    4. STANDARDS FOR ANESTHESIA: THE ISSUES   59
   Leslie Rendell-Baker, M.D.

SECTION 2. USING WHAT WE KNOW TO DESIGN FOR THE FUTURE   87

    5. COMPONENTS OF THE SYSTEM: FUTURE DESIGN REQUIREMENTS   89
   Jerry M. Calkins, Ph.D., M.D., and
   Reynolds J. Saunders, M.D.

6. GAS AND VAPOR DELIVERY   99
   Jerry M. Calkins, Ph.D., M.D., Reynolds J. Saunders, M.D., and Charles K. Waterson, B.S.E.

7. RECOVERY OF WASTE ANESTHETIC GASES   109
   Charles K. Waterson, B.S.E.

8. CONTROL OF ANESTHETIC DELIVERY   125
   Kenneth C. Mylrea, Ph.D.

9. MONITORING SYSTEM GAS CONCENTRATIONS   137
   Jerry M. Calkins, Ph.D., M.D.

10. GETTING THE DATA: REDUCING CONFUSION WITH THE COMPUTER   149
    Donald G. Schultz, Ph.D., and Walter J. Arnell, Ph.D.

11. ANESTHESIA VENTILATORS: SPECIAL REQUIREMENTS   165
    Charles W. Otto, M.D.

SECTION 3.   PROTOTYPES FOR THE FUTURE   175

12. THE ALABAMA AUTOMATED CLOSED-CIRCUIT ANESTHESIA PROJECT   177
    Jeffry A. Spain, M.D., Thomas C. Jannett, M.S., and Edward A. Ernst, M.D.

13. THE ARIZONA PROGRAM: DEVELOPMENT OF A MODULAR, INTERACTIVE ANESTHESIA DELIVERY SYSTEM   185
    Warren R. Jewett, Sc.D.

14. THE BOSTON ANESTHESIA SYSTEM   207
    Jeffrey B. Cooper, Ph.D., and Ronald S. Newbower, Ph.D.

15. THE UTAH SYSTEM: COMPUTER-CONTROLLED ANESTHETIC DELIVERY   221
    Dwayne R. Westenskow, Ph.D., and William S. Jordan, M.D.

SECTION 4.   THE FUTURE LIES AHEAD   235

16. WHAT DO WE DO UNTIL THE FUTURE GETS HERE?   237
    Reynolds J. Saunders, M.D.

INDEX   245

SECTION III

PROBLEMS AND CONTROVERSIES IN ANESTHETIC DELIVERY

Long gone from the contemporary anesthesia scene are the days of a cloth and an ether bottle. Present-day anesthesia apparatus are formidable, to say the least, and intimidating to the operator, at worst. Does complexity by necessity breed safety? What does the future hold in this technical area?

The first section of this issue is devoted to present capabilities, limitations, and future speculations concerning delivery of anesthetics and oxygen. There is no question that equipment design—state of the art—will not remain static. Change is inevitable. However, empiric reasoning dictates that design changes are complicated by the absolute requirement to demonstrate that new and more sophisticated technology is superior to contemporary technology. Integration of new concepts, such as computers and microprocessors, into anesthesia circuitry will occur. "Multitudinous functions permit multitudinous failures" is the other side of the coin, however. From an industrial engineering point of view, many advances and safety increases can be accomplished by better interfaces between anesthetist and machine. For several years, there has been a revival of closed-circuit anesthesia techniques. This renaissance has been due to increased understanding of uptake and distribution of the inhalation anesthetics. The technique has much to commend it, and it has been given a tremendous boost by new sensing and monitoring advances. The authors in this first section enthusiastically state their rationales for improved anesthesia delivery systems.

The first chapter answers the question, why new delivery systems? Chapter 2 discusses the advantages and disadvantages of open- and closed-circuit delivery systems. The third chapter presents an explanation of computers and how they work and explores the possible benefits of computer technology to the anesthesiologist. But chaos could reign if the geometric proliferation of new equipment, sensors, monitors, computers, dials, and whistles were to grow like Topsy. There must be standardization. The last chapter of this section discusses this important aspect of new equipment design and utilization.

Burnell R. Brown, Jr.

WHY NEW DELIVERY SYSTEMS?
Jerry M. Calkins, Ph.D., M.D.

WHY HAS NEW TECHNOLOGY SKIPPED ANESTHESIA?

Today's routinely used standard anesthesia machine is an excellent example of simple, reliable, traditional technology. In its simplest form, the anesthesia machine is a system composed of interconnected parallel sections of tubing and flowmeters that enables the user to produce an oxygen/nitrous oxide mixture at a desired concentration. To this mixture of gases is added a variable concentration of an anesthetic vapor. The resultant mixture is supplied to a breathing circuit and thence to the patient.

The basic anesthesia machine design has not changed significantly from the closed-circuit unit first described and built in 1914.[1] The successful application of this classic, 70-year-old design makes any improvement upon these proven techniques difficult. Further amelioration in performance using current technology cannot be accomplished easily without noticeable changes in cost, complexity, and reliability.[2]

Given successfully proven, mature design technology, why is it necessary that anesthetists embrace new, sophisticated design concepts, which may complicate a reliable technique of anesthesia delivery? Many anesthetists have emphasized this by stating, "I have not needed changes or additions to my equipment in my 20 years of practice. Why do I need them now?"

Although the reluctance for change on the parts of both anesthetists and manufacturers increases the frustration in the scientific community, it precludes the use of fads by limiting anesthesia delivery systems to proven, essential techniques which have stood the scrutiny of medical science. As a result, both the anesthesia and industrial communities find themselves in a Catch 22: there are not sufficient data to justify development of machines and instruments, nor are the machines and instruments necessary to obtain the data available.

Reluctance to redesign anesthesia systems is not unique to current thinking. After a demonstration of the reuse of nitrous oxide by means of a new rebreathing system employing a carbon dioxide absorber, the addition of carbon dioxide removal was not readily accepted; this led the developer to state that "the profession was just not yet ready for the closed system with carbon dioxide absorption."[1]

Similar analogies can be made to blood pressure measurement and the ECG, which are now widely utilized. Initially patients' blood pressures were measured using a Riva Rocci apparatus. Although economical, the technique was not convenient. Though it was more precise than feeling the pulse, routine application of the technique had not proven itself a necessity. Adoption of the method did not result from either the mystical aura of "science" or from fear that omission would lead to law suits. Acceptance probably resulted from the fact that the technique provided data that went beyond the normal senses, that is, it could signal a potential danger that might be influenced by the actions of the operator and of the anesthetic system.[3,4] Even the introduction of the ECG in anesthesia took a similar path: like blood pressure, the ECG data were not directly acquired by the senses. Likewise, it, too, had the potential to signal dangers and to be affected by the anesthetic and other operative procedures.[3,4]

WHY NEW DESIGNS?

Those who question the need and reasons for change in anesthesia delivery systems require justifiable answers prior to accepting and implementing new concepts which might be construed as "re-inventing the wheel." The reasons for new anesthesia delivery system designs are complex, interrelated, and multifaceted, stemming primarily from needs created by advances in medical and physiologic knowledge. Advances in medical technology have made it possible to make use of this new knowledge through complex regimens of care of the surgical patient. These advances have resulted in complex systems for postoperative monitoring and therapy. Because the period of greatest stress and instability usually occurs during anesthesia, an equivalent level of sophistication and automation is imperative in the delivery of anesthesia, particularly in those patients who already present great challenges in clinical management. However, in addition to the need for more sophisticated and precise patient care, pressures exist in the areas of medical/legal requirements, federal regulation, and cost effectiveness. Increasing patient safety through reduction of the risk of human error and machine hazards requires that the medical and manufacturing communities reassess product quality and efficacy in clinical situations.

Medicolegal considerations (critical incidents inciting litigation) have placed into perspective the importance of precluding exposure to liability by either eliminating or reducing the sources of liability, namely, injuries to surgical patients undergoing anesthesia.[5] Improvements in basic biomedical technology and the burden of increasingly stringent medicolegal requirements for surveillance and documentation of care have, in addition to these areas, increased the complexity of anesthesia delivery systems. This documentation of care has expanded to include the complexities of information gathering and surveillance monitoring, decision making, intervention, and record keeping.

Federal agencies such as the Food and Drug Administration have demanded—and rightly so—that prior to the introduction of new techniques, safety and efficacy be successfully demonstrated. Examining the device classification process reveals that older technologies, although licensed under "grandfather clauses," would not come close to meeting today's regulatory requirements and standards. Awareness of these deficits also adds a burden to the anesthesia community.

Cost effectiveness, with appropriate risk/benefit and benefit/cost ratios, also must be clearly demonstrated. With current rates of increase in medical costs, economic advantages of design changes in anesthesia delivery must clearly be demonstrated. One major area that has such data is the gas cost comparison between anesthetic delivery techniques. The improved economics of closed circuit or low flow systems versus the higher flow techniques support improvement in application and equipment. From measurement and calculation, no less than $80 million in gases (oxygen and nitrous oxide) were wasted via high flow techniques in the United States in 1977.[6] It is obvious that the cost is much higher when volatile anesthetic agents are considered. These losses must be passed on to the patient (and eventually to society).

The economic impact of widespread use of adequate low flow systems may be debated. However, the argument for improved patient care and safety through the reduction of critical mishaps resulting from equipment failure or human error is difficult to refute. Human error was believed to be a factor in 87 percent of 80 deaths,[7] 65 percent of 52 deaths,[8] and 83 percent of 589 deaths[9] attributed to anesthesia. From a data base of 790 preventable mishaps at four hospitals, investigators found that nearly 89 percent were attributable to human error.[10] Included are accidental disconnections of breathing circuits, intravenous tubing, and the like. Of these mishaps, only the remaining 11 percent were equipment failures, of which only a small percent of the mechanical failures were produced by malfunctions of the anesthetist's machine. Further analysis of these data indicated that 26 percent of the mishaps occurred during induction, 42 percent through the middle of the procedure, and only 9 percent at the end of the procedure. About one third of the human errors were found to be related to interactions between the breathing circuit and the anesthesia machine.[10]

Close observation of the anesthetist in action intuitively leads the observer to conclude that an appreciable risk exists from equipment per se and the complex interfacing of anesthetist, equipment, and patient. In addition to the previous studies, a limited number of studies to identify characteristics of interfacing problems and equipment-related risks have begun. One report considered certain aspects relating to the interfacing of anesthetist and machine. A significant finding of this study indicates that between 40 and 50 percent of the time in all operations the anesthesiologist is not involved in gross physical activity.[11] More recent investigators have studied the time and motion relationships between the mechanical and visual activities of the anesthesiologist.[12] Like the former study, these results indicated a distinct contrast between visual and manual activities. Approximately 60 percent of the visual activity involves patient and surgical field, and the remaining 40 percent of visual activity is directed elsewhere. The anesthetic period was divided into quarters, and the frequency of each type of activity was calculated for each quarter. Although manual activity occurred throughout the anesthetic procedure, the most active times occurred during the first and fourth quarters and the least activity during the third. A number of investigators have suggested that analogous stress and decision-making situations exist for both anesthesiologists and pilots.

The analogy between the anesthesiologist and the airplane pilot is appropriate.[3] Both must respond to changing situations. Both must interpret various forms of data and act to make necessary changes and corrections, and both are subjected to varying degrees of stress. Anesthesia can be administered without instruments, just as airplanes may be flown without a compass, but not for long periods or in adverse conditions.[3] Whether a reduction in stress would be beneficial to the anesthesiologist has not been demonstrated.

From the collective results of these and other studies, one can easily conclude that the design of anesthesia delivery systems, with appropriate interfacing among anesthetist, system, and patient, is far from optimal. It is quite evident the anesthetizing work area needs to have better definition, arrangement, and integration of control and information display units. This task must be accomplished in such a manner as to meet the specific needs of the work area, taking into consideration variability between individuals and situations.

WHAT NEW TECHNOLOGY IS AVAILABLE?

Since the whys for the delays in new designs and design concepts have been discussed, what new technologies are available for incorporation into these new delivery systems? Which technologies will add to the sophistication of the design without significantly increasing complexity and cost?

If anesthesia delivery is to modernize, then automation—including data acquisition and processing—is clearly the direction of the future. Because of the very nature of anesthesia delivery, the design will require both mechanical and electronic components with the necessary interfacing capabilities. This implies mechanical-electronic hybrid systems that employ the unique advantages of versatility and the economic benefits of each. The mechanical technology of fluidics and the electronic technology of solid state microelectronics appear to ideally "fit the bill."

Fluidics

Fluidics is defined by the National Fluid Power Association as "engineering science pertaining to the use of fluid dynamic phenomena to sense, control, process information, and/or actuate."[13] The word itself was derived from combining the two words fluid and logic. The field of fluidics includes pneumatics (fluidics with moving parts) and fluerics (fluidics without moving parts).

Because the anesthesia delivery system utilizes flowing gases and vapors, applications of fluidics are naturally appropriate. The technology for accurate flowmeters, concentration sensors, proportionating systems, ventilators, scavengers, and humidifiers exists. The main design problem is the integration of fluidic components with electronic microprocessors and controllers.

Microelectronics

With the current explosion in solid state microelectronics, the rapid development toward automation throughout industry is moving at a rapid pace. The focus of both this electronic technology and the designs of future delivery systems is the microcomputer and the necessary components to interface it with other subsystems. The microprocessor will enable the acquisition, processing, and unambiguous display of data that has been previously denied to the anesthetist. These advances will not remove the anesthetist from head of the table any more than the automatic pilot removed the pilot from the airplane.

SUMMARY

Although anesthetists have accomplished a remarkable safety record with commercially available anesthetic machines, these results have been obtained in spite of machine design, which could best be described as a nonsystem. In cases involving severely compromised patients, surgical procedures that severely alter patient physiology, and untoward events during "routine" anesthesia, it is a tribute to the flexibility and resourcefulness of anesthetists that more incidents do not occur. Industry has long sought precision, reliability, automatic control, and human-factors engineering in nonmedical applications, such as aircraft cockpit design, word-processing stations, and manufacturing processes. The relentless accretion of more and more nonintegrated gadgets onto an antiquated technology has exceeded the boundaries of proper function. Neither the patient nor the anesthetist is being served well by failure to implement state-of-the-art technology in anesthesic delivery systems. Anesthesiologists and others who are vitally interested in the welfare of their patients must insist that development of radically new integrated modular systems proceed at full speed. Their checkbooks can speak as loudly as the facts; it is time the manufacturers are aware that deep concern will be translated into purchasing decisions.

REFERENCES

1. JACKSON, DE: *Anesthesia equipment from 1914 to 1954 and experiments leading to its development.* Anesthesiology 16:953–969, 1955.
2. REAM, AK: *New directions—the anesthesia machine and the practice of anesthesia* (editorial). Anesthesiology 49:307–38, 1978.
3. GRAVENSTEIN, JS: *As for pilots, instruments important.* Engineering in Medicine and Biology 1:23–24, 1982.
4. GRAVENSTEIN, JS: *Failure to monitor.* In Gravenstein, JS, Newbower, RS, Ream, AK, Smith, NT, (EDS): *Essential Noninvasive Monitoring in Anesthesia.* Grune & Stratton, New York, 1980, pp 305–310.
5. DORNETTE, WHL: *Equipment-related injuries: Risks and safety factors.* Legal Perspectives on Anesthesia 1:5, pp 1–3, 1981.
6. LOWE, HJ, ERNST, EA: *The Quantitative Practice of Anesthesia. Use of Closed Circuit.* Williams & Wilkins, Baltimore, 1981.
7. DRIPPS, RD, LAMONT, A, ECKENHOFF, JE: *The role of anesthesia in surgical mortality.* JAMA 178:261–266, 1961.
8. CLIFTON, BS, HOTTEN, WIT: *Deaths associated with anesthesia.* Br J Anaesth 35:250–259, 1963.
9. EDWARDS, G, MORTON, HJV, PASK, EA, ET AL: *Deaths associated with anesthesia: Report on 1000 cases.* Anesthesia 11:194–220, 1956.
10. COOPER, JB, NEWBOWER, RS, LONG, CD, MCPEEK, B: *Preventable anesthesia mishaps: A study of human factors.* Anesthesiology 49:399–406, 1978.
11. DRUI, AB, BEHM, RJ, MARTIN, WE: *Predesign investigation of the anesthesia operational environment.* Anesth Analg 52:584–591, 1973.
12. BOQUET, G, BUSHMAN, JA, DAVENPORT, HT: *The anaesthetic machine—a study of function and design.* Br J Anaesth 52:61–67, 1980.
13. WHAT YOU SHOULD KNOW ABOUT FLUIDICS. Thiensville, WI, National Fluid Power Association, 1972.

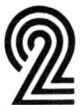

CLOSED-CIRCUIT AND HIGH-FLOW SYSTEMS: EXAMINING ALTERNATIVES

Edward A. Ernst, M.D., and
Jeffry A. Spain, M.D.

Every anesthesiologist has successfully used a high-flow system for the delivery of anesthetic drugs and oxygen during general anesthesia. How can the efficacy of such a system be questioned? For decades millions of patients have received safe anesthesia with high-flow nonrebreathing and partial rebreathing systems. Why should a total rebreathing, or closed, system even be considered as an alternate method of delivery?

Nothing is all good, totally advantageous, or beyond criticism. No anesthesia delivery system is perfect. Closed-circuit systems purport to solve many problems associated with open-circuit systems and, in addition, augment noninvasive monitoring capabilities. The purpose of this chapter is to look objectively at the advantages and disadvantages of open- and closed-circuit delivery systems and to draw conclusions from current knowledge and experience.

DEFINITION OF DELIVERY SYSTEMS

Traditionally, anesthesia delivery systems have been classified as open, semiopen, semiclosed, and closed, depending upon components of the delivery circuit: directional valves, reservoir, carbon dioxide absorber, and exhaust valve.[1] A simpler and more useful classification, proposed by Hamilton,[2] uses the required total delivery flow rate to define the type of system.

As seen in Table 1, closed-circuit anesthesia requires a *unique* delivery flow rate. Provided there are no leaks in the system, patient uptake determines the exact amount of gas that can be delivered into the system. Because there are no exhausted gases, delivered flows must equal patient uptake. If delivery rate exceeds patient consumption, the reservoir bag increases in size and eventually exceeds its capacity. If the rate of delivered gases is less than patient consumption, the reservoir decreases in size and eventually empties. In a closed circuit, individual patient uptake defines for the anesthesiologist the rate of delivery into the system.

Because closed circuit requires total rebreathing, a carbon dioxide absorber in the circuit is essential. Directional valves in the inspiratory and expiratory limbs of a circle system and a reservoir are also required (Fig. 1).

A nonrebreathing system requires the highest delivery flow rates because none of the exhaled gas is reinhaled. Figure 2 illustrates the classical Ayre's T-piece as a simple means of delivering anesthesia. The popular Bain system is functionally similar. Adding two valves to the system allows decrease of the delivery rate to the patient's minute ventilatory volume.

A partial rebreathing system is created when the delivery flow rates are less than those required for a nonrebreathing system and more than the amount permitted for a closed system. To prevent accumulation of exhaled carbon dioxide, a carbon dioxide absorber must be in the circuit. Unidirectional valves and a reservoir are needed, and a partially opened pop-off valve exhausts delivered gases in excess of patient uptake.

Table 1. Anesthesia Systems Classified According to Delivery Flow Rates

Type of System	Required Total Delivery Flow Rates
Closed	
total rebreathing	Patient uptake ($O_2 \simeq 1/24\ \dot{V}$)
Open	
nonrebreathing	$1\ \dot{V}$ to $3\ \dot{V}$ (minimal)
partial rebreathing	An infinite number of flows $> 1/24\ \dot{V}$ and $< 3\ \dot{V}$

$\dot{V}$ = patient minute ventilatory volume

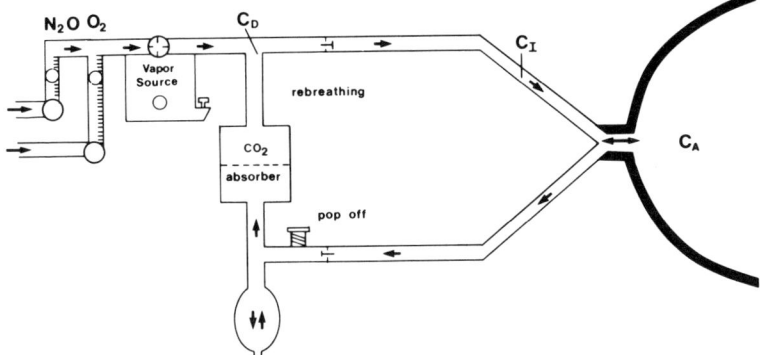

Figure 1. Diagram of a standard anesthesia circuit connected to a patient. It can be used as a closed (total rebreathing) or open (nonrebreathing or partial rebreathing) system, depending completely upon the rate of delivered gases. Except in a nonrebreathing system, delivered concentration (C_D) does not equal inhaled concentration (C_I), which in *any* case does not equal alveolar concentration (C_A).

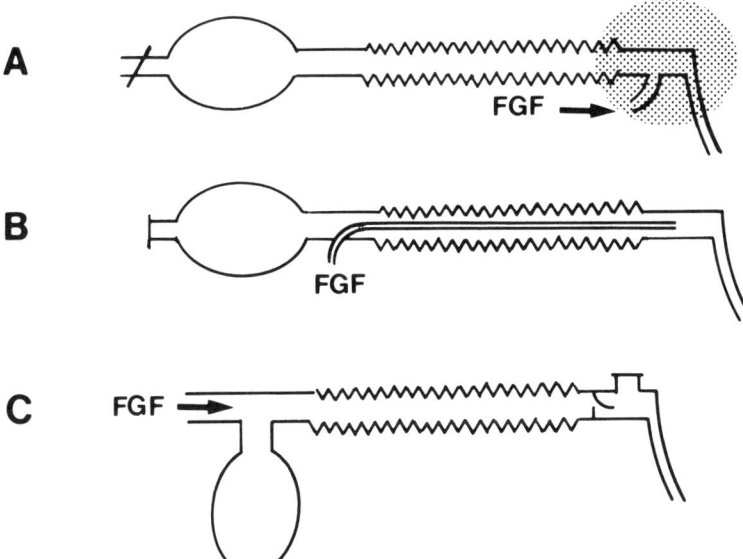

Figure 2. Nonrebreathing systems. *A*, classical Ayre's T-piece (shaded) modified with a reservoir on the exhalation port. Fresh gas flow (FGF) must exceed $1 \times \dot{V}$ to prevent rebreathing of exhaled CO_2. *B*, Popular coaxial Bain system functionally same as modified Ayre's. *C*, Addition of inspiratory and expiratory valves permit FGF to be reduced to $1 \dot{V}$.

ADVANTAGES AND DISADVANTAGES OF NONREBREATHING SYSTEMS

Perhaps the most important factor sustaining the popularity of nonrebreathing systems is that the concentration of gases delivered from the machine equals the inhaled concentration. By observing gas flows and vaporizer settings, the anesthesiologist has a fairly accurate knowledge of anesthetic and oxygen concentrations introduced into the lungs, breath by breath. Furthermore, the anesthesiologist can increase or decrease those concentrations very rapidly. In addition, the delivery system is simple and reliable. Stripped to its essential elements, the Ayre's system is simply a tube with a hole in it.

Nonrebreathing systems deliver up to 10 times the amount of drug required by the patient. Enteral or parenteral administration of drugs in such excessive quantities would have disastrous effects. Excessive gases and vapors are successfully administered because of their unique solubility characteristics. The amount of any gas that will dissolve in a given volume of liquid is limited, regardless of the volume of gas overlying the liquid or the length of time it is present. This physical property allows the anesthesiologist to deliver 5,000 ml per minute or more of 1 percent halothane, or any other desired concentration of anesthetic, into a system for hours and still administer perfectly safe anesthesia. What cannot be absorbed is vented through the pop-off valve.

The nonrebreathing system is the most inefficient of all systems. Efficiency is defined as:

$$\text{efficiency} = \frac{\text{amount of patient uptake}}{\text{amount delivered}}$$

In a hypothetical healthy 50 kg patient one hour into the anesthetic with 2,000 ml oxygen and 3,000 ml nitrous oxide being delivered per minute and the vaporizer set at 1 percent halothane (50 ml vapor), efficiency might be

for halothane,

$$\text{efficiency} = \frac{12.5}{50} = 0.25$$

for oxygen,

$$\text{efficiency} = \frac{200}{2000} = 0.10$$

and for nitrous oxide,

$$\text{efficiency} = \frac{125}{3000} = 0.04!!$$

Major disadvantages of the nonrebreathing system are related to the large quantities of vented gases. Eighty percent or more of the delivered gases are wasted. Herscher and Yeakel[3] conducted a study in which they recorded the amount of anesthetic agents introduced into high-flow circle systems used in their operating rooms and then measured the volume and concentration of gases exiting from the pop-off valves. From these data they calculated the amount of gases wasted during the study. Extrapolation of these data indicated a probable loss of $80 million in 1977 in the United States because of the predominant use of open systems. Edsall[4] challenged the economic advantage of closed circuit, stating that the additional cost of soda lime negated any financial gain. Spain[5] and others refuted Edsall's analysis, asserting that the total savings were substantial in the first hour and increased more as the anesthetic continued (Table 2). Calculated savings per 10,000 anesthetics, assuming 60 percent of the

Table 2. Material Costs (Dollars/Hr) for Open and Closed Anesthetic Systems Compared*

Agent	Open (Every Hour)	Closed			Cumulative Savings†	
		1st hr	2nd hr	3rd hr	Dollars	Percent
Halothane	0.89	0.51	0.27	0.24	1.89	62
Enflurane	4.14	2.13	0.86	0.69	8.74	70
Isoflurane	6.32	2.63	1.03	0.82	14.48	76

*70 kg healthy patient. Costs include 65% N_2O, 35% O_2, 0.65 MAC volatile agent (total MAC = 1.3), and, for closed system, soda lime
†after 3 hours with a closed circuit

anesthetics last one hour, 30 percent last two hours, and 10 percent last three hours, would be halothane $6,930, enflurane $36,670, and isoflurane $63,560. It is estimated that over 20 million anesthetics are given annually in the United States.

The cost advantage from anesthetic agents pales when compared with potential cost and energy savings that could be realized if the currently used no-return ventilating systems in operating rooms were converted to return systems. Basic code requirements published by the US Department of Health and Human Services, the Joint Commission on Hospital Accreditation, and other regulatory agencies provide guidelines for the ventilation of operating rooms. Total circulation rates vary from 15 to 25 air changes per hour. This rapid turnover is required to exhaust airborne contaminants affecting sterile conditions, to create proper air pressure differentials between sterile and nonsterile areas, and to exhaust excess anesthetics. Operating rooms are usually designed to utilize 100 percent outside air systems, exhausting everything into the atmosphere. Although effective bacterial filters exist, anesthetic agents, especially nitrous oxide, are ineffectively removed. If there were no anesthetic contaminants, operating room ventilating systems could return a high percentage of the heated or cooled air, thereby conserving a large amount of energy and netting a cost advantage.

Besides increasing cost, nonrebreathing systems pollute the operating room. The scavenging of waste anesthetic gases merely transfers them from the operating room to another environment, the atmosphere. Warnings that human activity might seriously reduce the earth's protective layer of ozone were first sounded in the early 1970s. Small amounts of ozone in the stratosphere, a region extending from about 15 to 60 kilometers above the earth's surface, play a vital function in screening out much of the sun's ultraviolet light, thus protecting plants and animals from harmful effects of high-energy radiation. Most ozone forms when sunlight strikes diatomic oxygen molecules:

$$O_2 \rightarrow O + O$$
$$O_2 + O \rightarrow O_3$$

The Rowland-Molina hypothesis states that fluorocarbons attack ozone. According to the hypothesis, chlorine can participate catalytically in the cycle and break down ozone:

$$Cl + O_3 \rightarrow ClO + O_2$$
$$\underline{ClO + O \rightarrow Cl + O_2}$$
$$O + O_3 \rightarrow 2O_2 \text{ net}$$

Uncertainties remain in the chlorofluorocarbon ozone-depletion hypothesis, but the Environmental Protection Agency (EPA) has attempted to limit such emissions in the United States. Anesthesiologists are not the only ones who use fluorocarbons.[6] In fact, they use a very small amount compared with industry. The federal government has imposed regulations in the last few years to drastically reduce fluorocarbon production for propellant and refrigerant use. Waste anesthetic gases may very well interest the EPA in the near future.

It is no secret that the National Institute of Occupational Safety Hazards (NIOSH) believes that trace anesthetic gas concentrations in operating rooms constitute an occupational hazard. Standards have arbitrarily been set and enforced. The maximum concentrations allowed for halothane, enflurane, and isoflurane are 0.5 parts per million, and for nitrous oxide it is 25 parts per million.[7] The only recommended solution has been scavenging devices, but they are costly, frequently fail, and have even been associated with intraoperative death.[8] In addition, NIOSH standards require that a comprehensive preplacement medical and occupational history be obtained and maintained in employees' medical records and that this information be updated at least yearly. Annual physical exams are required, and any abnormal outcome of pregnancy must be documented. The records must be maintained for a period of 20 years after termination of employment. Anesthesiologists are encumbered with federal regulations, threats, and restrictive conditions as a result of high-flow anesthetic systems.

In addition to the financial and environmental disadvantages of the open system, a few physiologic problems may be associated with it when anesthetic gases are not humidified before delivery to the patient. The compressed gases, nitrous oxide and oxygen, flow through reducing valves and must be "bone dry" to prevent the valves from freezing and obstructing flow. In an intubated patient, functionally deprived of turbinates, the cilia and lining of the trachea are the first structures to receive this arid onslaught. The gases are immediately heated to body temperature and saturated with water by the first mucous membrane encountered, resulting in dehydration and loss of ciliary action. The insult is increased during nonrebreathing anesthesia because none of the exhaled water or heat is reinhaled. Equipment is available for artificial heating and humidification of the inhaled gases, but, unfortunately, it is not generally employed.

PARTIAL REBREATHING SYSTEMS AND THEIR PROBLEMS

Some of the disadvantages of nonrebreathing systems are decreased by the use of a partial rebreathing system: less drug is used, less drug is exhausted from the system, and less water and heat are lost from the patient. The magnitude of these advantages is directly related to the degree of decreased delivery flow rate.

Partial rebreathing systems, sometimes referred to as semiclosed systems, constitute a vast no man's land between nonrebreathing and total rebreathing systems. The two extremes of flow rates are identified by the closed system on one hand and by the nonrebreathing system on the other. In partial rebreathing systems, some of the exhaled gas must be recycled in order to satisfy the minute ventilation. Many different flow rates can be used for partial rebreathing systems, and the amount of vapor emitted from the pop-off valve during various flow rates is impossible to assess.

The lower flow rates are responsible for the advantages and, concomitantly, the disadvantages. Because the rebreathed gas usually contains a different concentration than the fresh gas inflow, the inhaled concentration cannot equal the concentration of gas delivered by the gas machine. The anesthesiologist no longer knows with any degree of certainty the inhaled concentration

With all open systems the gases flowing into the delivery system have two fates: They can be absorbed by the patient and components of the delivery system or exhausted from the pop-off valve. Everything exhausted is wasted, contributes to pollution, and currently needs to be scavenged. Because the amount wasted is not measured, it is impossible to determine the amount of uptake of anesthetic agent or oxygen by the patient.

CLOSED-CIRCUIT SYSTEM

Closed-circuit anesthesia answers the objections to open systems related to high-delivery flow rates: cost, pollution, efficiency, and the hydration of inhaled gases. Table 2 compares drug and material costs. In addition, the possibility of eliminating scavenging systems is attractive. Closed-circuit anesthesia provides a means of controlling unwanted emissions *at their source.* Efficiency for anesthetic agents and oxygen is 1.0 because the delivered amount must equal the patient's uptake for the circuit to remain closed.

However, all these advantages are insignificant compared with the noninvasive physiologic and pharmacologic monitoring capabilities provided by closed-circuit anesthesia. Because delivery of oxygen from the gas machine must equal patient uptake, minute-oxygen consumption can be read from the oxygen flowmeter. The anesthesiologist then has a precise knowledge of the patient's oxygen consumption and related transport and metabolic variables such as carbon dioxide production, fluid requirement, and cardiovascular and respiratory performance. *Finally, the gas machine itself becomes a monitor!*

Monitoring Advantages

During closed-circuit anesthesia, the anesthesia machine becomes a pulmonary and cardiovascular function laboratory at the head of the table. Measured variables, unique to closed-circuit anesthesia, include patient minute-oxygen uptake, accurate tidal volume and dynamic compliance, and amount of anesthetic agent uptake. Calculated variables include basic fluid requirement as a function of oxygen consumption, carbon dioxide production and the necessary ventilation to provide any desired partial pressure of carbon dioxide in the arterial blood ($PaCO_2$), and directional changes in cardiac output. Degree of diaphragmatic myoneural junction paralysis is monitored noninvasively.

COMPARISON OF PREDICTED AND MEASURED OXYGEN CONSUMPTION

Brody[9] has shown a linear logarithmic correlation between oxygen consumption and weight in kilograms. In mammals of all sizes, from mice to elephants, oxygen consumption in ml per min equals $10.15 \times$ weight $(kg)^{0.73}$. For practical purposes, the equation is rounded off to 10 $kg^{3/4}$. This function is an excellent predictor of oxygen consumption at basal conditions, and a basal state is induced during anesthesia. If the patient is overweight, a correction should be made to acknowledge the low metabolic rate of fat.[10] Abernethy and coworkers[11] used the Metropolitan Life equation to determine patients' degree of fatness. He determined variations from ideal body weight (IBW) calculated as 110 lbs for males and 100 lbs for females $\pm$ 5 lbs per inch above or below 5 feet height.

If predicted oxygen consumption is compared with that measured during closed-circuit anesthesia, attempts to explain variations from predicted values may lead the anesthesiologist to deduce changes in cardiac output or metabolic rate. As can be seen from Figure 3, the amount of oxygen uptake is related to cardiac output, minute ventilation, carbon dioxide production, and basal fluid requirements. According to the Fick principle, oxygen consumption is the product of cardiac output and arterial-venous (a-v) oxygen difference. Since the a-v difference is fairly constant, except in severe pathologic states, trends in cardiac output can be estimated from measured oxygen uptake. A decrease in oxygen uptake should be considered related to a decrease in cardiac output until proven otherwise.

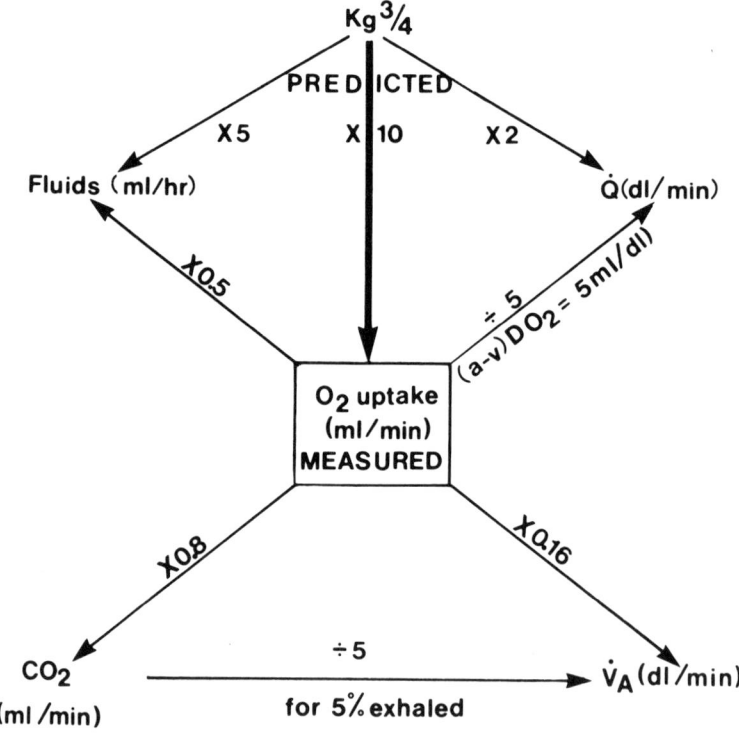

Figure 3. Patient weight ($kg^{3/4}$) as a predictor of metabolic and transport variables. Measured O_2 uptake is related to cardiac output ($\dot{Q}$), fluid requirements, CO_2 production, and minute alveolar ventilation ($\dot{V}_A$) required to maintain any desired Pa_{CO_2}.

Assuming an average respiratory quotient (RQ) of 0.8, individual carbon dioxide production can be calculated from the measured oxygen uptake. Furthermore, the alveolar ventilation necessary to excrete the minute carbon dioxide production can be predicted. For a $PaCO_2$ of about 38 mm Hg, an alveolar concentration of 5 percent carbon dioxide is necessary at sea level. The alveolar minute volume (V_A) can be determined in that case by dividing the minute carbon dioxide production by 5. By adding the estimated dead space, an accurate total minute volume can be predicted for any $PaCO_2$ desired.

Even fluid requirements are determined by oxygen consumption. Fluids are primarily used to excrete the waste products of aerobic metabolism, especially heat by evaporation. As indicated in Figure 3, the basal fluid requirement in ml per hr can be predicted by multiplying the measured oxygen use by 0.5.

The current metabolic state of the patient is revealed partially by oxygen consumption. Clinically, it is reassuring to measure a normal intraoperative oxygen uptake during a hypotensive episode. Normal oxygen consumption indicates that an oxygen debt is probably not developing. If oxygen consumption decreases under such conditions, the need for resuscitative measures is urgent. The success or failure of resuscitation is reflected by the measured oxygen consumption. Variations in body temperature are immediately reflected by changes in oxygen consumption, but acute episodes of hyperthyroidism and malignant hyperthermia have been first detected by a change in oxygen uptake well before changes in pulse, skin color, and temperature occurred.

QUANTITATIVE PULMONARY DYNAMICS

Accurate tidal volumes can be measured via the gas reservoir bag or ventilator bellows because excessive gases are not flowing into the system and disrupting the change in reservoir size during ventilation. High flow rates buffer the reservoir's displacement and rate of movement. The Ventimeter ventilator illustrated in Figure 4 is used as the reservoir, and its spirometer bellows measures tidal volume during spontaneous, assisted, or controlled ventilation.

More important, exhalant flow rates can be measured. Exhalation is completely patient dependent, and the exhalation flow rate is decreased with bronchospasm, air trapping, and other pathologic conditions. Exhaled flow rates can be decreased to a degree at which exhalation is not complete before the next inhalation begins, despite an extremely slow respiratory rate. The use of a spirometer ventilator

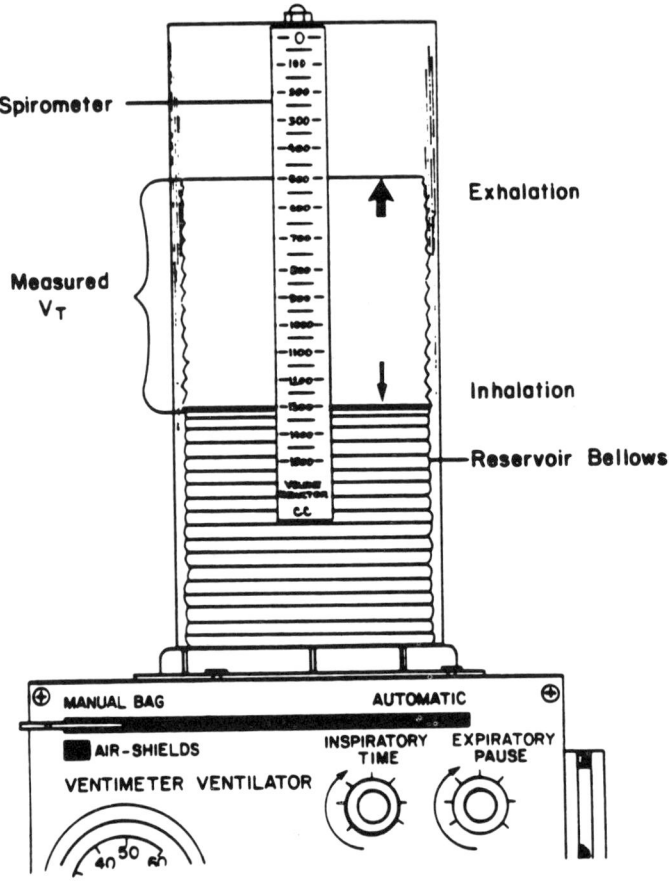

Figure 4. Schematic of upright bellows ventilator. The spirometer measures accurate tidal volumes during closed-circuit anesthesia because there is no excessive fresh gas flow to influence bellows movement. Fresh gas flow must be adjusted so that the bellows does not rise to the top of the ventilator, causing the pop-off valve to open. (Adapted, with permission, from Narco Scientific/Air-Shields Division, Hatboro, Pa.).

in a closed circuit reveals such a clinical condition. This information is lost when the bellows rapidly rises owing to the high inflow rate of fresh gas.

At the end-tidal phase of respiration, slight movements of the spirometer bellows reflect changes in intrathoracic volume. The stroke volume of each heartbeat is frequently seen in the form of a slight bellows excursion coincident with the cardiac cycle. In a completely paralyzed patient, one of the earliest indicators of additional relaxant need is a slight diaphragmatic motion sensitively displayed by movements of the spirometer bellows. The diaphragm recovers well before the extremity muscles conventionally monitored by peripheral nerve stimulators. Titration of additional muscle relaxant drugs results in the disappearance of diaphragmatic motion, as revealed by quiescence of the spirometer bellows. The reservoir becomes another noninvasive monitor, following the degree of myoneural junction block.

Because accurate tidal volumes are measured, pulmonary dynamic compliance (change in volume/change in pressure) can be accurately followed breath by breath. Anesthetic uptake problems associated with dead space, seen in open systems, are minimal when a closed system is used. This is because all gases except carbon dioxide are rebreathed.

Problems and Concerns

Practitioners accustomed to high-flow systems voice two major concerns about closed-circuit anesthesia: "I have the feeling that it is unsafe, and it certainly might be in my hands" and "It would require that I pay too much attention to mathematics and machinery and less attention to my patient." Both concerns are legitimate and must be adequately answered before closed-circuit anesthesia can be safely practiced. The answer to the first concern lies in education. To that end, a textbook on the topic has been published,[10] two international symposia have been held, and articles in refereed journals concerning closed-circuit anesthesia are numerous. Clinical tutorials are offered at some teaching institutions. The answer to the second concern will require the development of better anesthesia machines that are leakproof, will accurately meter gases at low flow rates, and can monitor circuit concentrations. Such equipment is well along in its development.

SPECIFIC CONCERNS AND RESPONSES

A hypoxic mixture may be delivered. This is true. It is also true when a high-flow system is used. Hypoxic brain damage following anesthetic procedures is a major cause of lawsuits today. A reliable, well-maintained oxygen analyzer should monitor circuit gases during all anesthetics regardless of the type of system used. This is monitoring at the consumer level. Anesthesiologists say, "I don't trust an oxygen analyzer." That is good. The anesthesiologist should not trust anything but should constantly monitor the patient clinically, reinforcing information provided by mechanical or electronic sources. Should we trust a flowmeter? An ECG machine? A manometer? Or the numerous other instruments that constantly aid us in the practice of anesthesia?

Another method of assuring adequate inhaled oxygen concentration is to use a system using only one gas: oxygen. The use of only oxygen does not absolutely excuse the anesthesiologist from employing an oxygen analyzer. It has happened that technicians inadvertently switched oxygen and nitrous oxide inlet lines on gas machines used later by anesthesiologists unaware of the mistake, resulting in patient death. Some anesthesiologists may be concerned about oxygen toxicity if oxygen only is used. If such a concern exists, it is a simple matter to introduce nitrogen in the form of air into the closed breathing circuit at any time during the anesthetic, keeping the oxygen concentration at any desired level.

An unsafe concentration of anesthetic agent may be delivered. That is true. And, of course, it is also true with open systems. Regardless of the delivery system, the anesthesiologist is not excused from monitoring the patient's depth of anesthesia. During closed-circuit anesthesia the amount of agent delivered into the system must be adjusted, just as the successful clinician adjusts delivery concentrations during an open system. It is not necessary to adhere to a "square root of time" model or any other model to effectively practice closed-circuit anesthesia. It can be done empirically. If the circuit concentration of the anesthetic agent is monitored with an EMMA, Narcotest, mass spectrometer, or other instrument, the delivery of anesthetic agent is made even simpler.

It is not essential to know a sophisticated uptake and distribution model in order to successfully practice closed-circuit anesthesia. Most anesthesiologists learned the technique of open-circuit anesthesia before mastering uptake and distribution principles. They were told to deliver 1 percent (or other concentration) halothane, or 2 percent enflurane, and to adjust the delivery concentration according to patient response. Similar empiricisms are applicable to closed-circuit delivery.

The concentration of nitrogen will increase in the system. It cannot be a problem if the patient's lungs are adequately denitrogenated prior to closing the system. Barton and Nunn[12] have shown that the concentration of nitrogen increases about 4 percent in a closed circuit after 80 minutes if the patient's lungs have been adequately denitrogenated. This is not a surprising finding. The total amount of nitrogen dissolved in fat and water in the usual adult patient is about 1 liter. The volume of gas into which this liter of nitrogen could escape is about 10 liters, the sum of the circuit's volume of 7.5 liters and the patient's functional residual capacity of 2.5 liters. This analysis shows that the maximal increase in circuit nitrogen would be limited to about 10 percent.

Dangerous levels of carbon monoxide, methane, or other volatiles will accumulate in the system. These have not been found to be clinically important. However, these and other gases have been measured during closed-circuit anesthesia and found to increase. More carbon monoxide is found in smokers than nonsmokers. Hydrogen, acetone, and methane increase, approaching flammable levels in some patients.[13] To date, no patient has been reported harmed from rebreathing exhaled volatiles, but this is an interesting finding and one which should be followed closely. If accumulation of volatile substances in a closed circuit is shown to be important, it may be necessary to empty the breathing bag occasionally and to provide fresh gas.

It requires leakproof equipment, calibrated flowmeters, accurate vaporizers—all maintained in excellent condition. This should be true of all anesthesia equipment, regardless of the system used. In this day of high technology, the number of equipment faults the anesthesiologist will accept is remarkable. Does the machine leak? "What difference does it make? I can compensate for the leak by simply increasing the flows." Are the flowmeters accurate? "Who cares? With the high flow rates I am using, there is little difference between 4,000 and 5,000 ml of oxygen per minute." Anesthesiologists have been trained to check their machines for leaks and then to proceed to create the greatest leak of all through the pop-off valve. In an era of control technology and precision, we encourage imprecision through the use of high-flow systems. It is time anesthesiologists demand the best in quality equipment to practice their precarious trade.

Closed-circuit anesthesia invites additional medicolegal risks. Closed-circuit anesthesia is not considered an experimental procedure. For a decade it was used for the administration of cyclopropane, long before the square root of time theory or the use of oxygen analyzers. No plaintiff has brought suit against an anesthesiologist because of closed-circuit use. On the contrary, Mazzia and Simon[14] have predicted that anesthesiologists might be brought to court for *not* using closed-circuit anesthesia should a pollution-related health problem occur among operating room personnel.

The depth of anesthesia cannot be readily decreased, and the patient cannot quickly emerge from anesthesia without opening the system. This was a serious criticism of closed-circuit anesthesia before the utilization of a charcoal shunt to filter inspiratory gases during emergence.[15] By diverting gases through a charcoal filter placed in the inspiratory limb of the circuit (Fig. 5), the inhaled concentration of volatile anesthetic agents becomes undetectable and the level of anesthesia is lightened at a maximal rate. It has always been possible to increase closed-circuit concentrations very rapidly, and the use of the charcoal filter now allows a very rapid decrease in circuit concentration during closed-circuit anesthesia.

Figure 6 displays inspiratory and expiratory concentrations of halothane as monitored by a mass spectrometer at the endotracheal tube. Activation of the charcoal shunt rapidly brings the inspiratory concentration to zero, despite the continuation of a closed-circuit system.

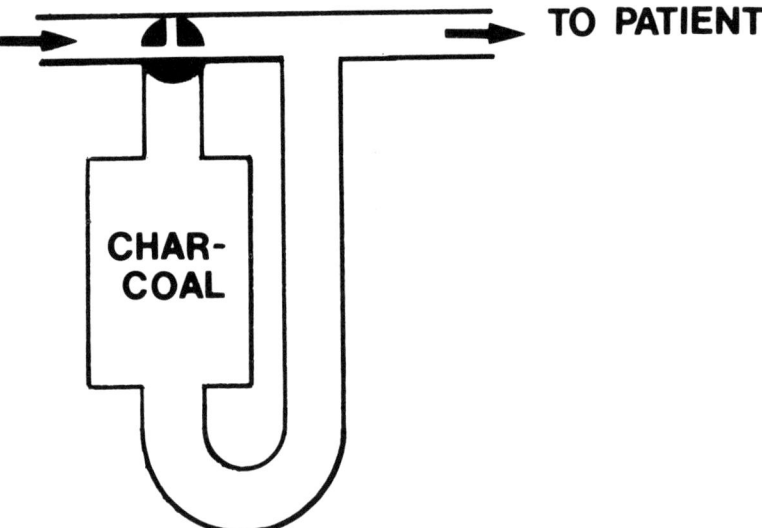

Figure 5. Charcoal shunt adaptation placed on the inspiratory limb of an anesthesia circuit. Turning the valve 90° forces all inspiratory gases through the charcoal, producing a 0 inhaled concentration of any volatile anesthetic agent.

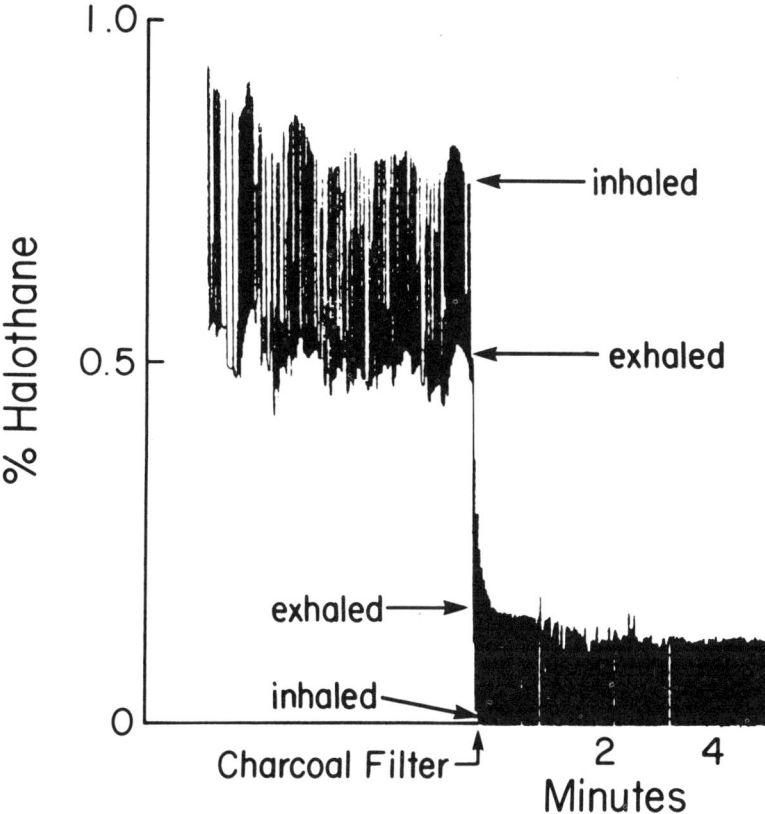

Figure 6. Mass spectrometer recordings of inhaled and exhaled halothane concentrations after 2 hours of halothane anesthesia as detected from the endotracheal tube. Prior to the onset of charcoal filtration, the exhaled concentration was 0.5 percent halothane (above movement threshold for the patient). Turning on the charcoal filter brought the inspiratory concentration to 0 within three breaths, and the patient responded to commands within 4 minutes.

Fifty grams of charcoal will adsorb 2000 ml of halothane vapor before any halothane is detectable in the exhausted gas. This provides at least 30 minutes of use during emergence, and most patients awaken at about 11 minutes following a 2-hour halothane anesthetic.

Charcoal is safe and has been used in gas masks for decades. It adsorbs all volatile anesthetic very rapidly and efficiently but adsorbs nitrous oxide poorly.[16,17] Dry charcoal adsorbs more volatile agents than wet charcoal, and resistance to gas flow through it is negligible. Charcoal need not be discarded after use and can be reactivated by autoclaving.[18]

Clinical Practice

"BALANCED" ANESTHESIA

The simplest and easiest way to become acquainted with closed-circuit anesthesia is to employ it during a narcotic-relaxant-nitrous oxide-oxygen anesthetic, a so-called balanced anesthetic. An in-circuit oxygen analyzer and initial pulmonary denitrogenation are mandatory. The same schedule of analgesics and relaxants is kept as with an open system, the pop-off valve is closed *after pulmonary denitrogenation,* and the flows of nitrous oxide and oxygen are reduced so that the reservoir bag does not overdistend or empty. The flows of nitrous oxide and oxygen must be adjusted to satisfy two conditions: The breathing bag reservoir must fill to about the same degree at end-tidal exhalation, and the circuit oxygen concentration must remain nearly constant at a desired level. Table 3 lists the conditions and methods of control.

USE OF VOLATILE ANESTHETICS

Another condition is required when using volatile agents in a closed circuit. The circuit concentration of the volatile agent associated with a desired level of anesthesia must be attained and maintained. Table 4 tabulates considerations for the additional condition.

By what means are volatile agents introduced into a closed circuit, and in what amount? Safe deliveries using a Tek type vaporizer, copper kettle, liquid injection, and in-circuit vaporizer have been described.[10] Tables displaying recommended doses are published

Table 3. Conditions to be Maintained during Closed-Circuit "Balanced" Anesthesia

Conditions	How Measured	How Controlled
Constant circuit volume	End-tidal volume of breathing bag reservoir	Adjustment of O_2 and N_2O flows in the same direction
Constant circuit O_2 concentration	O_2 analyzer	Adjustment of O_2 and N_2O flows in opposite directions

Table 4. Additional Condition to be Maintained during Closed-Circuit Volatile Anesthesia Administration

Condition	How Measured	How Controlled
Proper circuit volatile agent concentrations	1. Clinically 2. Circuit analyzer	Introduce agent 1. Tek vaporizer 2. Copper kettle 3. Liquid injection in circuit 4. In-circuit vaporizer Extract agent 1. Charcoal filter

(see Tables 5 and 6). Any *predicted* dose is just a starting point and must be *adjusted* according to individual patient response—just as the delivered concentration into an open system is adjusted. Adjustments are made according to the clinical response of the patient and, if available, the measured circuit concentration.

The decrease in uptake, as time goes on, requires that less and less anesthetic agent be delivered into the circuit. One way of decreasing the delivered amount is to increase the intervals at which a certain predicted or recommended dose is given. Uptake and distribution the-

Table 5. Standard Unit Dose for 0.65 MAC

Patient Wt (kg)	Halothane		Isoflurane		Enflurane	
	ml liq	ml O_2/min[†]	ml liq	ml O_2/min[†]	ml liq	ml O_2/min[†]
40	0.31	159	0.39	165	0.64	430
50	0.37	188	0.46	194	0.75	509
60	0.42	216	0.53	223	0.86	583
70	0.47	242	0.60	250	0.97	655
80	0.52	268	0.66	277	1.07	724
90	0.57	293	0.72	302	1.17	791
100	0.62	317	0.78	327	1.26	856
110	0.66	340	0.84	351	1.36	919
120	0.71	363	0.89	375	1.45	981
130	0.75	386	0.95	398	1.54	1042

[†]O_2 flow through copper kettle vaporizer to deliver unit dose in 1 minute

Table 6. Tek Settings for 0.65 MAC

Elapsed Time (Hr:Min)	Elapsed Time (Min)	Time Interval (Min)	Vaporizer Dial Setting (%) (ml/dl or Volume %)		
			Halothane	Isoflurane	Enflurane
0:00	0	1	4.6	4.9	7.0
0:01	1	3	3.9	4.2	7.0
0:04	4	5	3.4	3.6	7.0
0:09	9	7	2.9	3.2	7.0
0:16	16	9	2.6	2.8	5.2
0:25	25	11	2.4	2.5	4.1
0:36	36	13	2.1	2.3	3.8
0:49	49	15	2.0	2.1	3.5
1:04	64	17	1.8	2.0	3.2
1:21	81	19	1.7	1.8	3.0

ory suggests that the administration intervals increase sequentially by 2 minutes each. In other words, if 0.31 ml of liquid halothane is required in the first minute, then, theoretically, the same amount should be required during the next 3 minutes, then the next 5 minutes, then the next 7 minutes. Many closed-circuit practitioners, however, simply adjust the delivery rate according to individual patient response. The recommended Tek settings predicted to maintain 0.65 the minimal alveolar concentration (MAC) volatile agent when 65 percent nitrous oxide is used are displayed in Table 6. The Tek settings are also changed at time intervals increasing by 2 minutes each.

Injecting liquid volatile agent into the exhalation limb of a circuit may seem risky to those not familiar with the technique. After all, the concentration of halothane at the site of injection is about 33 percent. However, when diluted in the circuit volume the inhaled concentration can be 1 percent, 2 percent, or any other desired concentration, depending upon the amount injected.

The injection technique represents the ultimate vaporizer. A precisely known amount of vapor is delivered into the circuit with each injection. Calibration is never a problem. The total amount of anesthetic used can be read from the syringe at any time. Tek type vaporizers have been shown to deliver different concentrations of agent when different concentrations of nitrous oxide flow through them.[19] Also, output concentrations may vary unpredictably with carrier gas flow rate.

The use of a charcoal filter shunt makes it possible to lighten the anesthetic during the procedure, if desired, and to awaken the patient at the end of the procedure. Without this device, it is necessary to open the circuit and to use high flows of oxygen during emergence.

Theory

During closed-circuit anesthesia, delivered gases have only one fate. The pop-off valve remains closed, and all delivered gases must be absorbed by the patient or by the delivery system. The task of the closed system practitioner is to be able to predict the amount of anesthetic needed to attain and to maintain a proper anesthetic level. Is there a clinically useful model by which such a prediction can be made?

UPTAKE PREDICTIONS USING THE ZÜNTZ EQUATION

The relationship defining the rate at which individual organs take up anesthetic agents was originally described by Züntz[20] in 1897:

$$\dot{Q}an_o = Ca\dot{Q}_o e - \frac{\dot{Q}_o t}{V_o \lambda_{T/B}}$$

where Ca is the arterial concentration, $\dot{Q}_o$ the organ blood flow, V_o the organ volume, $\lambda_{T/B}$ the tissue/blood partition coefficient, and t the elapsed time.

This relationship states that initially an organ takes up the anesthetic agent at the rate at which it is delivered by arterial blood ($Ca\dot{Q}_o$). As time goes by, this rate falls off exponentially, like radioactive decay, with a time constant or half-life directly proportional to the capacity of the organ for the agent ($V_o \lambda_{T/B}$), and inversely proportional to the organ blood flow ($\dot{Q}_o$). The arterial concentration (Ca) is assumed to be constant.

The rate of uptake of anesthetic agent by the whole body ($\dot{Q}an_T$) can be calculated by summation of the uptakes of each individual organ or tissue given by the Züntz equation. Each organ will, of course, be characterized by different values of $\dot{Q}_o$, V_o, and $\lambda_{T/B}$ giving each a different time constant of uptake rate decay:

$$\dot{Q}an_T = Ca\dot{Q}_{o1}(\text{exponential 1}) + Ca\dot{Q}_{o2}(\text{exponential 2})$$

$$+ \cdots + Ca\dot{Q}_{on}(\text{exponential n})$$

At time zero, all exponential terms have the value of 1, so the initial rate of anesthetic uptake by the whole body is as follows:

$$Qan_T \text{ at time zero} = Ca\dot{Q}_{o1} + Ca\dot{Q}_{o2} + \cdots + Ca\dot{Q}_{on}$$

Because Ca, for anatomical reasons, is the same for all organs, and since the sum of all the individual organ blood flows ($\dot{Q}_o$) is equal to the cardiac output ($\dot{Q}$), the initial rate of whole body anesthetic uptake can be written as

$$\dot{Q}an_T \text{ at time zero} = Ca\dot{Q}$$

This rate will fall off with time in a complex fashion related to the combination of all the exponential decay terms for the individual organs.

Several authors, including Eger,[21] have computed numerical solutions for the rate of whole body anesthetic uptake. However, the computational burden is too great to make the Züntz relationship useful for the prediction of anesthetic uptake in clinical practice.

UPTAKE PREDICTIONS USING THE SQUARE ROOT OF TIME MODEL

The square root of time model was first described by Severinghaus[22] in 1952 for whole body uptake of nitrous oxide. In 1972 Lowe[23] delivered volatile anesthetic agents to patients using a closed circuit so that a constant arterial anesthetic concentration was maintained. In doing so he discovered that the square root of time model was valid for these agents as well.

The square root of time model is a very simple relationship which states:

$$\dot{Q}an_T = Ca\dot{Q}t^{-1/2}$$

where $t^{-1/2}$ is the reciprocal of the square root of the elapsed anesthetic time.

The simplicity of this equation makes it very useful in clinical practice.[24] Note that the square root of time relationship is similar in form to the Züntz relationship for whole body anesthetic uptake. Both have the term $Ca\dot{Q}$ in common. In the square root of time model, the term $t^{-1/2}$ approximates the rate at which whole body anesthetic uptake decreases with time.

The two models agree with each other remarkably well. Figure 7 shows the result of a computer simulation in which the kinetics of anesthetic uptake were modeled using the Züntz relationship for eight separate tissue compartments. In the simulation the anesthetic agent was delivered to the model using the square root of time equation for a desired arterial concentration of 1.3 MAC. If the two models had agreed exactly, the amount of agent delivered would have exactly equaled the amount taken up by the body, resulting in a constant arterial concentration of 1.3 MAC. The closeness of the predicted arterial concentration in the simulation to the desired concentration shows how well the square root of time model agrees with the classical Züntz model.

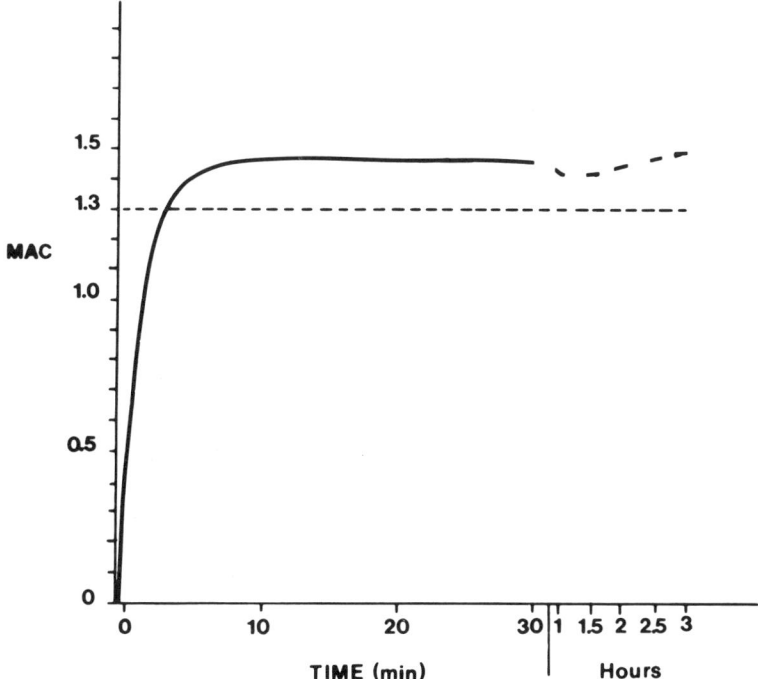

Figure 7. Computer simulation of total body halothane uptake for a 70 kg patient as predicted from the Züntz model. Halothane was administered according to the square root of time model to achieve a desired arterial concentration of 1.3 MAC. The solid line shows the predicted arterial halothane concentration as a function of time, and the dashed line shows the desired concentration, both over a 3-hour time period.

PRACTICAL USE OF THE SQUARE ROOT OF TIME MODEL

In the clinical practice of closed-circuit anesthesia it is more convenient to consider the cumulative dose of an anesthetic agent than its rate of uptake. This can be obtained by integration of the square root of time equation for uptake:

$$\text{Cumulative dose} = \int_0^t \dot{Q}an_T dt$$
$$= \int_0^t Ca\dot{Q}t^{-1/2} dt$$
$$= 2Ca\dot{Q}t^{1/2}$$

Assuming that Ca and $\dot{Q}$ are relatively constant, the term $2Ca\dot{Q}$ defines a unit dose of the anesthetic agent. The term $t^{1/2}$, the square root of the elapsed anesthetic time usually measured in $\sqrt{\text{minutes}}$, defines the time at which a unit dose should be administered. Figure 8 graphically illustrates the value of the unit dose concept. On the left side (A) the cumulative dose of halothane for a 100 kg patient is

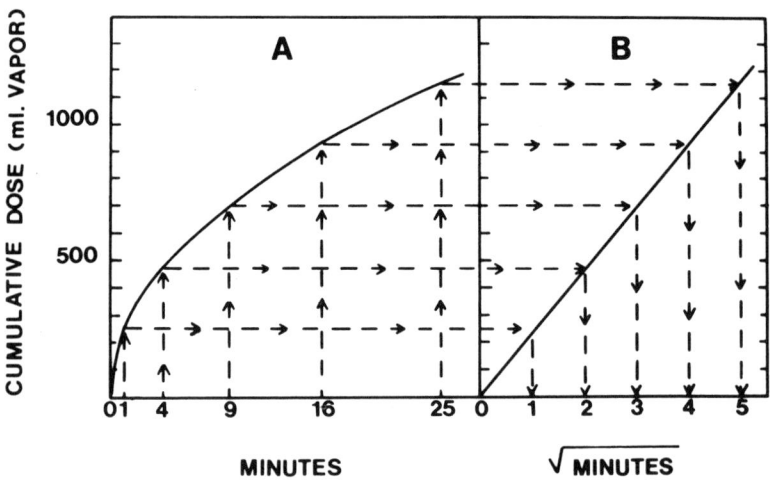

Figure 8. Cumulative uptake of halothane by a theoretical 100 kg patient as (A) a function of real time and as (B) a function of the square root of time. Note that the same amount of halothane is taken up during each square root of time interval.

Table 7. Reference Times

$t^{1/2}$ ($\sqrt{\text{minutes}}$)	0	1	2	3	4	5	6 ...
t (minutes)	0	1	4	9	16	25	36 ...
interval (minutes)		1	3	5	7	9	11 ...

plotted as a function of real time. The dosage curve becomes a straight line on the right side of the figure (B) when the cumulative dose is plotted against the square root of time ($\sqrt{\text{minutes}}$). Note that the same incremental one-unit dose of halothane is delivered after each square root of time interval. These times correspond to progressively longer intervals of real time as shown in Table 7. The intervals of real time form a sequence of consecutive odd integers and increase by 2 minutes each. In practice the predicted unit dose can be calculated in advance when the desired arterial concentration and the patient's weight are known. For 0.65 MAC halothane in a typical adult patient weighing 70 to 80 kg, the predicted unit dose is about 0.5 ml liquid (see Table 5) or 100 ml of vapor. It should be emphasized, however, that the model serves only as a guide in clinical situations. Although it works well most of the time, the anesthesiologist must adjust the dose of volatile anesthetic agent based on the patient's clinical status, just as for any other drug.

Determination of Unit Dose ($2Ca\dot{Q}$)

The unit dose can be calculated using the patient's weight and the anticipated desired alveolar concentration.

$$\text{Unit dose} = 2Ca\dot{Q} = 2 \underbrace{\underbrace{\underbrace{f\, MAC}_{C_A} \times \lambda_{B/G}}_{Ca} \times \dot{Q}}_{\text{minute arterial delivery } (Ca\dot{Q})}$$

unit dose

where f = fractional MAC desired, MAC = the minimal alveolar concentration, C_A = the alveolar concentration, $\lambda_{B/G}$ = the blood/gas partition coefficient for the agent used, Ca = the arterial concentration, and $\dot{Q}$ = the cardiac output ($2kg^{3/4}$ in dl per min).

Example: 100 kg patient ($\dot{Q} = 2 \times 100^{3/4} = 63.25$ dl per min)

1.3 MAC halothane-oxygen anesthetic anticipated

unit dose = $2 \times 1.3 \times 0.75 \times 2.4 \times 63.25$
= 296 ml halothane vapor
= 1.2 ml halothane liquid (1ml liq = 240 ml vapor)

One unit dose is administered during the first minute, during the next 3 minutes, and during the next 5 minutes.

In addition to the unit dose, the system must be primed at time 0. The prime dose is that amount of agent required to bring the breathing circuit and functional residual capacity to the desired alveolar concentration and to fill the arterial delivery system with the desired concentration. Ordinarily, as a first approximation, 1 unit dose can be used for the prime dose. For those who wish to calculate individual prime doses, the following formula is provided:

$$\text{prime dose} = \underbrace{C_a \dot{Q}}_{} + \text{Vvent} \times f\,\text{MAC}$$

$$= \underbrace{f\,\text{MAC} \times \lambda_{B/G}}_{C_A} \times Q + \text{Vvent} \times \underbrace{f\,\text{MAC}}_{C_A}$$

$$\underbrace{\hspace{5em}}_{C_a}$$

$$\underbrace{\hspace{8em}}_{\text{arterial prime}} + \underbrace{\hspace{6em}}_{\text{ventilatory prime}}$$

where Vvent = volume of anesthetic circuit and functional residual capacity.

As an example, the prime dose required by a 100 kg patient receiving halothane where $f = 1.3$, MAC = 0.75, Vvent = 100 dl, and $\dot{Q} = 2$ kg$^{3/4}$ (or 63.25 dl) is

halothane prime = $1.3 \times 0.75 \times 2.4 \times 63.25$
$+ 100 \times 1.3 \times 0.75$
prime dose = 246 ml of halothane vapor, or about 1.0 ml liquid

SUMMARY

The nonrebreathing system has been with us since Morton demonstrated the administration of diethyl ether in 1846. Its current popularity is evidenced by the extensive use of the Bain system. The greatest advantage, its history of patient safety, is related to the circuit's simplicity and the knowledge that the delivered concentration equals the inhaled concentration. Most disadvantages of the nonrebreathing system are related to the required high delivery rates: operating room and environmental pollution, necessity of scavenging gases, cost of agents, energy loss through no-return operating room ventilation, inhalation of dry gases, and the inability of the anesthesiologist to quantitate patient uptake of oxygen and inhaled anesthetics.

Partial rebreathing systems reduce the disadvantages related to high delivery flow rates but, owing to the required rebreathing, do not permit the anesthesiologist to know the inhaled anesthetic concentration. A carbon dioxide absorber is necessary. It is still impossible to quantitate uptake by the patient, and it is difficult to conclude that any real net advantage results from the use of partial rebreathing systems.

When modern-day technology provides the practitioner with an appropriate anesthesia machine, it is likely that closed-circuit anesthesia will become the method of choice for anesthesia delivery. Although the economic, ecologic, and physiologic advantages of this system are important, its greatest asset is the ability to monitor important respiratory and cardiovascular variables in patients noninvasively. Important information provided to the anesthesiologist by the patient during closed-circuit anesthesia is lost through the pop-off valve when high-flow systems are used. During closed-circuit anesthesia the gas machine itself becomes a monitor. Practicing anesthesiologists will embrace closed-circuit anesthesia practice when—and if—they are convinced that it provides an opportunity for better and more efficient patient care than other systems.

REFERENCES

1. MOYERS, J: *A nomenclature for methods of inhalation anesthesia.* Anesthesiology 14:609, 1953.
2. HAMILTON, W: *Nomenclature of inhalation anesthetic systems.* Anesthesiology 25:3, 1964.
3. HERSCHER, E AND YEAKEL, AE: *Nitrous oxide-oxygen based anesthesia: The waste and its cost.* Anesthesiology Review 4:29, 1977.
4. EDSALL, DW: *Economy is not a major benefit of closed system anesthesia.* Anesthesiology 54:258, 1981.
5. SPAIN, J: *Costs of delivery of anesthetic gases reexamined III.* Anesthesiology 55:711, 1981.

6. Fox, JL: Atmospheric ozone issue looms again. Chemical Engineering News, p 25, October 15, 1979.
7. *NIOSH criteria for recommended standards . . . occupational exposure to waste anesthetic gases and vapors.* Department of Health, Education and Welfare, Washington, DC, March, 1977.
8. Sharrock, NE and Gabel, RA: *Inadvertent anesthetic overdose obscured by scavenging.* Anesthesiology 49:137, 1978.
9. Brody, S: *Bioenergetics and growth.* Reinhold, New York, 1945.
10. Lowe, HJ and Ernst, EA: *The Quantitative Practice of Anesthesia—Use of Closed Circuit.* Williams & Wilkins, Baltimore, 1981.
11. Abernethy, DR, et al: *Alterations in drug distribution and clearance due to obesity.* J Pharmocol Exp Ther 217:681–685, 1981, p 147.
12. Barton, F and Nunn, JR: *Use of refractometry to determine nitrogen accumulation in closed circuits.* Br J Anaesth 47:348, 1975.
13. Morita, S, et al: *Accumulation of methane, acetone, and nitrogen in the inspired gas during closed circuit anesthesia.* Anesth Analg 60:267–268, April, 1981.
14. Mazzia, VDB and Simon, AH: *Legal liability and some specific cases.* In Aldrete, JA, Lowe, HJ, and Virtue, RW (eds): *Low Flow and Closed System Anesthesia.* Grune & Stratton, New York, 1979.
15. Ernst, EA: *In-circuit charcoal filter to rapidly reduce alveolar anesthetic concentration while maintaining a closed circuit.* Anesthesiology 57:343, 1982.
16. Maggs, FAP and Smith, ME: *Adsorption of anesthetic vapours on charcoal beds.* Anesthesia 31:30–40, 1976.
17. Kim, BM and Sircar, S: *Adsorption characteristics of volatile anesthetics on activated carbons and performance of carbon canisters.* Anesthesiology 46:159–165, 1977.
18. Capon, JH: *A method of regenerating activated charcoal anaesthetic adsorbers by autoclaving.* Anaesthesia 29:611–614, 1974.
19. Lin, CY: *Assessment of vaporizer performance in low-flow and closed circuit anesthesia.* Anesth Analg 59:359–366, 1980.
20. Züntz, N: *Zü pathogenese und therapie der durch rasche luft druck anderungen erzerzliegten krankheiten.* Fortschr Med 15:632, 1897.
21. Eger, EI II: *Anesthetic Uptake and Action.* Williams & Wilkins, Baltimore, 1974, p 89.
22. Severinghaus, JW: *The rate of uptake of nitrous oxide in man.* J Clin Invest 33:1183, 1954.
23. Lowe, HJ: *Dose-Regulated Penthrane Methoxyflurane Anesthesia.* Abbott Laboratories, Chicago, 1972, pp 85–87.
24. Spain, JA: *Computer assisted closed circuit anesthesia.* Anesthesiology (Suppl) 53:S366, 1980.

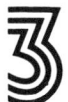

COMPUTERS: DO WE NEED THEM NOW?

Jeffry A. Spain, M.D., and
Reynolds J. Saunders, M.D.

In 1946 the first electronic digital computer became operational. The Electronic Numerical Integrator and Calculator (ENIAC) was built at a cost of several hundred thousand dollars using 18,000 vacuum tubes and 1,500 mechanical relays. It was able to perform about 1000 arithmetic calculations per second, and it filled a large room.[1] In the ensuing four decades we have witnessed an enormous growth of computer technology. The most powerful computers of today are built of tiny integrated circuit chips instead of vacuum tubes, and they can perform over 100,000,000 arithmetic calculations per second.[2] These computers still cost millions of dollars and fill large rooms, but today a device with the computing power of the ENIAC can be purchased for a few hundred dollars and held in the palm of one's hand.

The first electronic computers were used to help develop the hydrogen bomb, and succeeding generations of computers have continued to have a profound impact on our civilization. It is no exaggeration to say that today's society would collapse almost entirely if all computers suddenly disappeared. Paradoxically, most people have very little comprehension of the inherent capabilities and limitations of these devices on which we are so dependent. Over the past decade computer technology has begun to revolutionize the practice of medicine as well. Sophisticated monitoring and diagnostic equipment has been developed, of which computerized tomography is an obvious example. Some of the monitoring equipment used by clinical anesthesiologists in the operating room is now controlled by microprocessors—whole computers on a single integrated circuit chip.

There is a clear trend toward an increasing role for computers in the practice of medicine, particularly in anesthesiology. It therefore becomes imperative that we gain a more precise understanding of both computers and the processes of anesthesia delivery so that this role can be properly defined. The purpose of this chapter is to explain what computers are and how they work, to outline some of the processes of anesthesia delivery, and to discuss how computers and anesthesiology might be integrated.

THE STRUCTURE AND FUNCTION OF COMPUTERS

In functional terms digital computers are the same today as they were 40 years ago, and they are able to perform three basic tasks (Fig. 1). First they can take information from the external environment and store it internally. Then, with this information, computers can perform calculations and store the results. Finally the results can be given again to the external environment.

Here is an example to illustrate these principles. Suppose that an anesthesiologist wished to have a computer monitor a patient's heart rate and sound an alarm if the heart rate were outside certain limits. First the computer might take two numbers typed on a keyboard, say

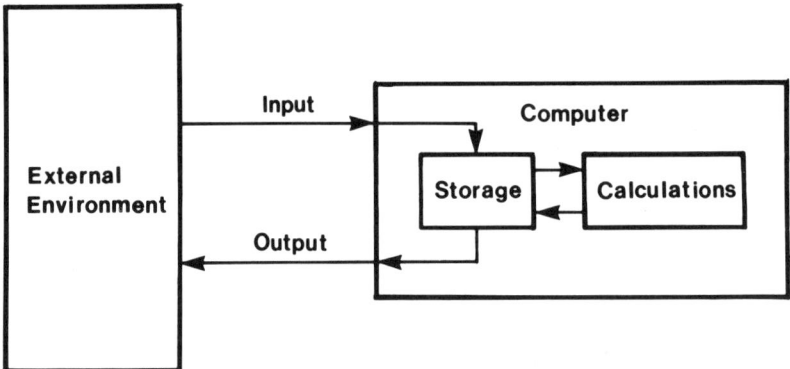

Figure 1. A basic functional block diagram of a digital computer. The boxes represent functional elements, and the arrows indicate the flow of information.

50 and 100, for use as the alarm limits. Then the computer would take the patient's heart rate from an ECG monitor connected to it and compare the heart rate data to the previously stored alarm limits. If the heart rate were less than 50 or greater than 100, the computer would give a command to turn on a buzzer. Otherwise the computer would turn off the buzzer. Then the computer would take another heart rate value from the monitor and repeat the process.

This example is obviously a trivial one, and it belies the sophistication that can be achieved. The computers on board the space shuttle Columbia, performing a large series of these same three basic tasks, are able to take information from navigational instruments aboard the spacecraft, calculate the flight path, and give commands to fire rockets and to move control surfaces. These computers literally fly the shuttle along its preprogrammed course.

The functions of input and storage, calculation, and output are built into digital computers according to design principles first expressed

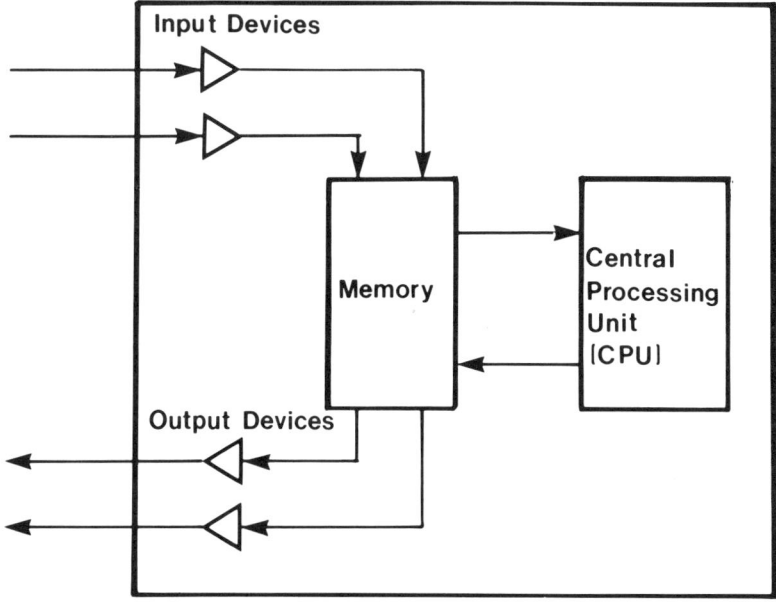

Figure 2. A basic structural block diagram of a digital computer. The boxes represent structural elements, the triangles signify interfaces between the computer and the external environment, and the arrows indicate the flow of information.

by John von Neumann and others at the Princeton Institute of Advanced Studies in 1946.[3] Almost all computers designed since then consist of three structural elements: input/output devices (I/O), a memory or storage area, and a central processing unit (CPU) (Fig. 2).

Input/Output Devices

Input/output devices connect computers to the external environment, and there are many different kinds of them, as one might expect from the complex nature of our world. Perhaps the most common I/O device today is the cathode ray tube (CRT) computer terminal. Information is put in from a keyboard, and "printed" characters are put out to a television screen. Other I/O devices include punched card and paper tape readers and punches, in which information is coded in the pattern of holes; printers, which imprint symbols on paper with an inked ribbon; plotters, which draw graphs by moving a pen; and magnetic disk and tape drives. Data are stored on a magnetic disk in a concentric circular pattern as the disk spins. Different circles—or tracks, as they are called—can be reached randomly by moving the recording head radially inward or outward. Digital magnetic tape drives store data serially along the tape just as analog tape decks record music.

The adjectives *digital* and *analog* are used frequently in discussing computers, and they require further explanation. These terms describe the form in which information is represented (Fig. 3). The word digital is derived from the Latin word for "fingers," as in counting on one's fingers. It implies that information is represented as a sequence of numbers, each of which has a discrete value within a certain range. The word analog is derived from the Greek word meaning proportionate. It implies that information is represented as a continuously varying signal, usually an electrical voltage, which at any given instant of time can have any value within a certain range. An example of an analog device is a cassette tape player that reads music in the form of a time-varying magnetic flux from the moving tape, generates an electrical analog of this signal, and finally uses the latter to drive a loudspeaker, which generates the equivalent acoustic signal, the sound of the music. Recently digital tape recorders for music have been introduced. Here the music is stored as a series of numbers on the tape. Successive numbers represent the sound pressure of the musical signal at successive moments in time. Perhaps

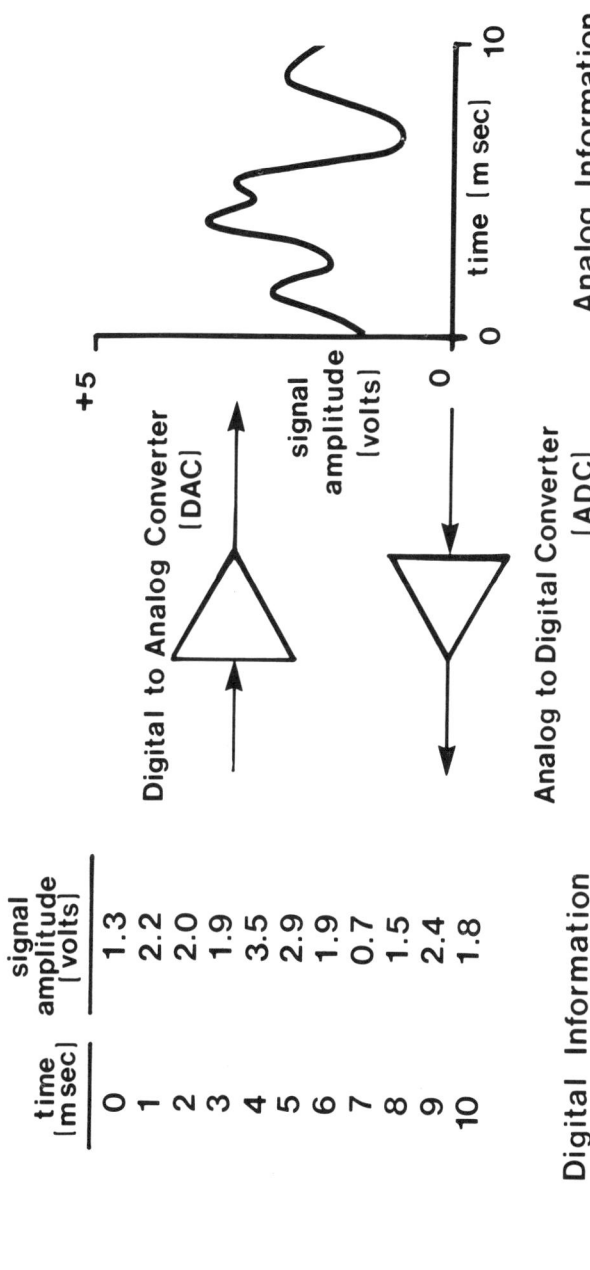

Figure 3. (*Left*) Digital and (*right*) analog representations of information. The (*center*) triangles symbolize converters between the two modalities.

COMPUTERS: DO WE NEED THEM NOW?

50,000 numbers would represent one second of music. To play the music, the numbers are read and converted sequentially to a time-varying analog voltage by a device called a digital-to-analog converter (DAC). This signal is used to drive the loudspeaker, and again music is heard.

In addition to DACs there are also analog-to-digital converters (ADCs). ADCs can sample a time-varying electrical voltage at successive instants of time and generate a sequence of numbers to represent the voltage. Because digital computers deal with information exclusively in digital form, DACs and ADCs give computers a great deal of versatility in interacting with the real world, in which almost all information is in analog form. The only remaining elements of this interaction not yet mentioned are transducers, which convert various forms of analog information into analog electrical signals and vice versa. For instance, loudspeakers transduce electrical signals to acoustic signals. Microphones reverse the process. Other such transducer pairs are light bulbs and photoelectric cells, television screens and video cameras, and servomotors and potentiometers for rotational motion, to name only a few. The strain gauge pressure transducer and thermistor temperature probe are two transducers commonly used in anesthesiology. In summary, all these devices easily can be interfaced with computers for the purpose of monitoring and controlling the outside environment.

Memory

The second essential element of digital computers is the storage area, or memory.* Here all the input data for calculations as well as the results of calculations are stored in the form of binary numbers. Binary numbers are composed of a sequence of digits called bits, each of which can have the value 0 or 1 (Fig. 4). Moving from right to left in a binary number, bits increase in significance by powers of two—we speak of the one's, two's, four's, and eight's place, and so on. Thus the number thirteen would be represented as 1101. In contrast, people generally calculate with decimal numbers that are composed of a sequence of digits, each of which can have the value 0 through 9. Moving from right to left in a decimal number, digits increase in signif-

---

*It is interesting to note that such anthropomorphic terms as *memory*, programming *language*, and even electronic *brain* are routinely applied to computers made of inanimate silicon and aluminum.

```
           8 + 4 + 0 + 1 = 13                      10 + 3 = 13
           ||  ||  ||  ||                           ||   ||
 ... 32 16  8   4   2   1         ... 1000  100    10    1
            x   x   x   x                           x    x
            1   1   0   1                           1    3
           BINARY SYSTEM                         DECIMAL SYSTEM
```

Figure 4. (*Left*) binary and (*right*) decimal representations of the number thirteen. The bottom row of numerals contains the bit or digit symbols for the two representations of the number thirteen, the middle row contains the place values (in decimal form) corresponding to the binary and decimal number systems, and the top row is the product of the bottom two rows in decimal form. The sum of the numbers in the top row shows the formation of the number thirteen in each case.

icance by powers of ten—we refer to the one's, ten's, hundred's, and thousand's place. The number thirteen is represented as 13.

Binary numbers are very convenient for computers to handle because each bit can have only two values. Thus computer memory circuits can be made of electronic switches that are set either on or off to represent a 1 or a 0. One key to the speed and compactness of today's computers is the fact that these switches typically can change state several million times per second and can be packaged as integrated circuits in which each switch occupies an area of only a few square micrometers. A typical microcomputer might have an internal memory capacity of just over half a million bits (Fig. 5). This memory is usually organized into cells of eight bits each, called bytes. Each byte of memory can store a number with any value between 0 and 255 inclusive, and each byte can be independently read and written by the computer. Occasionally the computer deals with half a byte at a time; this subunit is called a nybble. The location of each byte in memory is referred to as its address. Addresses are numbered sequentially from zero to some maximum, typically 64k for a microcomputer. Lowercase k is short for kilo, which means 1024, or 2^{10} here. A 64k byte memory contains $64 \times 1024 \times 8 = 524,288$ bits or switches. For example, the computer could store the number 119 at address 27592, and eight specific bits in the middle of the memory would be set to 01110111. The number previously stored at this address would be lost. Later, on one or more occasions, the computer could read address 27592 and retrieve the number 119. This type of memory is called random access memory (RAM). Another common type of memory is read-only memory (ROM). Addresses in ROM can be read but not written over or erased by the computer in normal oper-

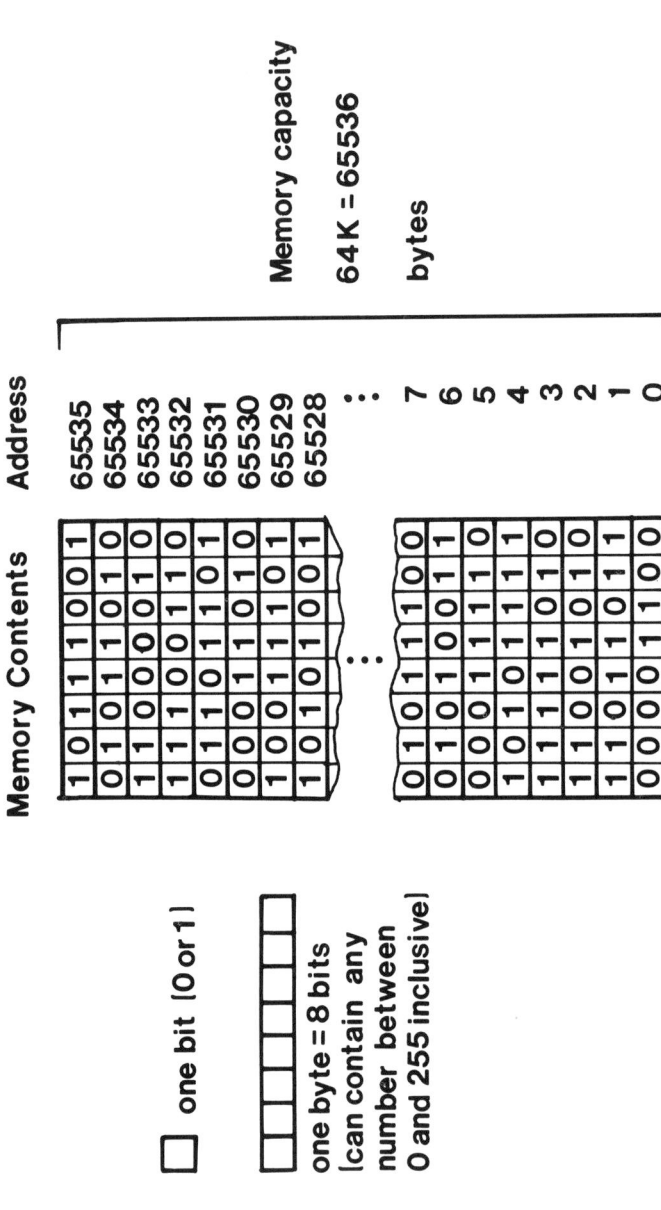

Figure 5. The internal memory of a microcomputer. Each small box represents one binary bit which may have a value of either 0 or 1. Eight bits form a byte, which may store a number with any value between 0 and 255 (decimal). The memory is organized as a sequence of bytes, each of which may be reached by a unique address.

ation. ROMs are generally used to store programs of which multiple copies are distributed to many users. Game cartridges for home video games contain ROMs in which the game programs are stored. In contrast to RAM, ROM does not "forget" what has been stored when its electrical power is turned off.*

In addition to internal RAM and ROM, computers usually have some form of external memory or mass storage. Mass storage devices are really a type of input/output device as well as a memory. The most common types of mass storage in use today are magnetic disk and tape drives. It is important to note that compared to RAM and ROM on integrated circuits, disks and tapes can store data at significantly higher densities and lower costs. A single 8-inch flexible diskette, which is commonly used with office word processors, can store about 1.2 million bytes, is smaller than a record album, and costs less than $10. The equivalent amount of RAM would occupy a space somewhat larger than a shoe box and cost over $10,000. Of course, there is another consideration, access time. The retrieval of a specific byte from a flexible diskette would require an average delay of 100 msec; RAM is about a million times faster. Magnetic tape is generally used for archival storage of infrequently used data. The data density is somewhat greater than that of disks, and the cost per byte is about one tenth as much. Tapes have significantly longer average access times owing to the fact that data are stored serially. To use two bytes at opposite ends of a tape, the computer must wind the entire tape through the drive.

The Central Processing Unit

The final structural element of computers to be discussed is the central processing unit (CPU). All the other I/O devices and memory units are linked to and controlled by the CPU, hence the term central. The CPU executes the basic tasks of input, calculation, and output according to a set of instructions called a program (Fig. 6).

The program is stored in sequential addresses in memory along with the data that it will manipulate during its execution. As von Neumann pointed out, this situation creates the possibility that a sophisticated program could modify its own instructions and hence "learn" from

---

*Another interesting device is the write-only memory (WOM). A WOM of unlimited capacity can easily be made from a small block of wood. WOMs and human memory often have strikingly similar characteristics!

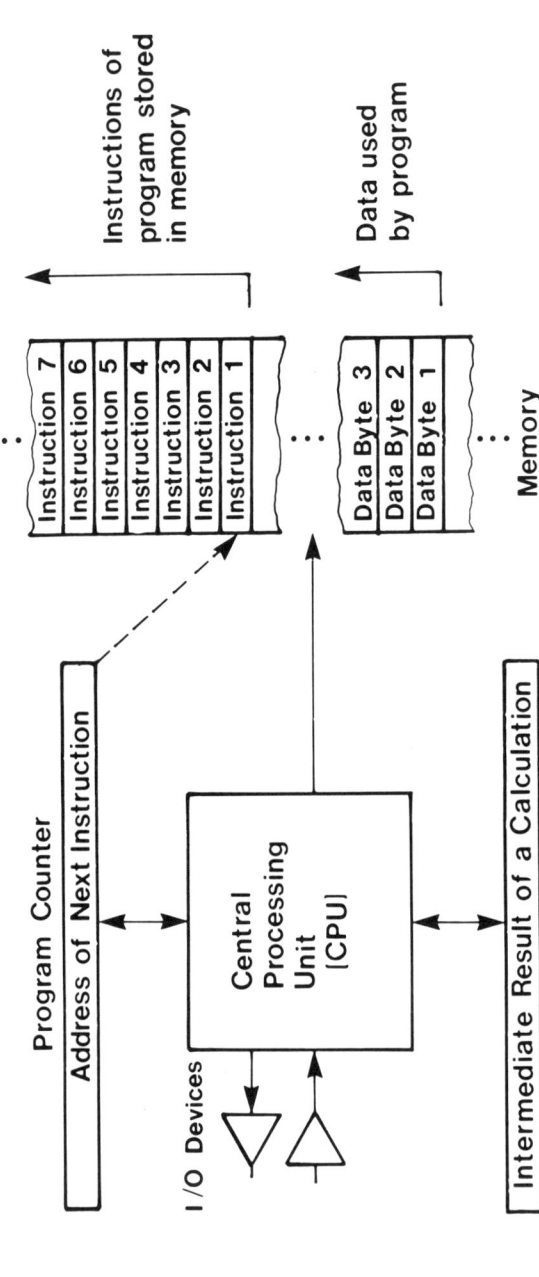

Figure 6. The execution of a program by the central processing unit. The program counter contains the memory address of the first instruction to be executed. Various instructions may cause the CPU to read or to write data bytes in memory. Intermediate results of calculations are stored in the accumulator.

experience. Usually, however, a program modifies itself only in circumstances unforeseen by the programmer, leading to an abrupt cessation of normal operation or "crash."

To execute a program, the CPU first looks at a special memory register called the program counter (PC). The PC contains the memory address of the next instruction of the program to be executed. The CPU then reads this byte of memory to find the binary code of the instruction. Next the CPU decodes the instruction and performs the specified operation. Note that although some instructions occupy only one byte of memory, others may require two or more to specify additional data pertinent to the execution of the instruction. These would be decoded in turn. Finally the PC is updated to point to the next instruction in sequence, and the cycle repeats. The CPU of a typical microcomputer can execute this instruction cycle about 500,000 times per second. This is an astonishingly rapid rate when one realizes that if a person working by hand could execute the same instructions at the rate of one every ten seconds, almost two months of continuous effort would be required to complete each 500,000.

Each instruction encodes a very specific command to the CPU. For example, one instruction might cause the CPU to input a number from an analog-to-digital converter and store it in the accumulator (ACC). The ACC is another special memory register internal to the CPU that is used to store data temporarily. Another instruction might add the contents of a specific memory location to the ACC. A third might store the contents of the ACC somewhere in memory or output the contents of the ACC to an I/O device. Instructions such as these are referred to generically as arithmetic and I/O instructions. A series of these instructions stored in consecutive memory locations would be executed by the CPU once through in sequence.

Another class of instructions, called control transfer instructions, allows the CPU to alter the sequence of instruction execution by modifying the program counter. These instructions confer real computing power on the CPU by allowing it to make decisions and to execute repetitively a segment of a program. For example, a control transfer instruction might cause the CPU to compare the contents of a specified memory location to the accumulator. If the values were equal, the program counter would remain unaltered; otherwise the CPU would load the program counter with another value specified in the instruction. In other words, if the two values were equal, the flow of the program would continue undisturbed. If they were unequal, control would jump to another section of the program. If one wanted to write a program to print a table of the square roots of the integers one through ten, the instructions to calculate the square root of a number and to print the result would need to be stored in memory only once. The CPU could be led to execute this code ten times, using the appropriate integer each time, through the use of control transfer instructions. The resultant saving of memory space, program size, and programming time should be evident.

PROGRAMMING

For a computer to execute a program, it must first be stored in the memory of the computer in binary number form. Translating a computing task into this form by hand and loading it into memory using console switches would certainly be unacceptably difficult, time-consuming, and error prone. Fortunately it is also unnecessary. Virtually all computers today are supplied with special programs called operating systems and language translators that vastly simplify this task.

An operating system is a program that facilitates the handling of other programs by a computer system (Fig. 7). The hardware of a typical microcomputer system might consist of a CPU, 64k bytes of memory, two flexible diskette drives, a printer, and a CRT terminal. In this case the operating system program is stored on a flexible diskette. When the system is turned on, the user presses a reset button on the console. Typically this causes the CPU to execute a program called the bootstrap loader, which is permanently stored in ROM. The bootstrap loader activates the flexible diskette drive, into which the operating system diskette has been placed, loads the operating system from the diskette into RAM, and transfers control to it. The operating system then displays a message on the CRT and waits for the user to type a command on the keyboard.

An operating system generally handles information in units called files. A file is a sequence of bytes of arbitrary contents and arbitrary length, limited only by the storage capacity of the system. A file might contain a program, a set of data, or the text of a document. Files are usually stored on diskettes, and the operating system keeps a name for each file and the file's location in a directory also stored on the diskette. Through the terminal keyboard the user can manipulate these files at will—creating them, modifying them, deleting them, copying them, and listing their contents on the printer. File creation and modification are done using an editing program. Here the contents

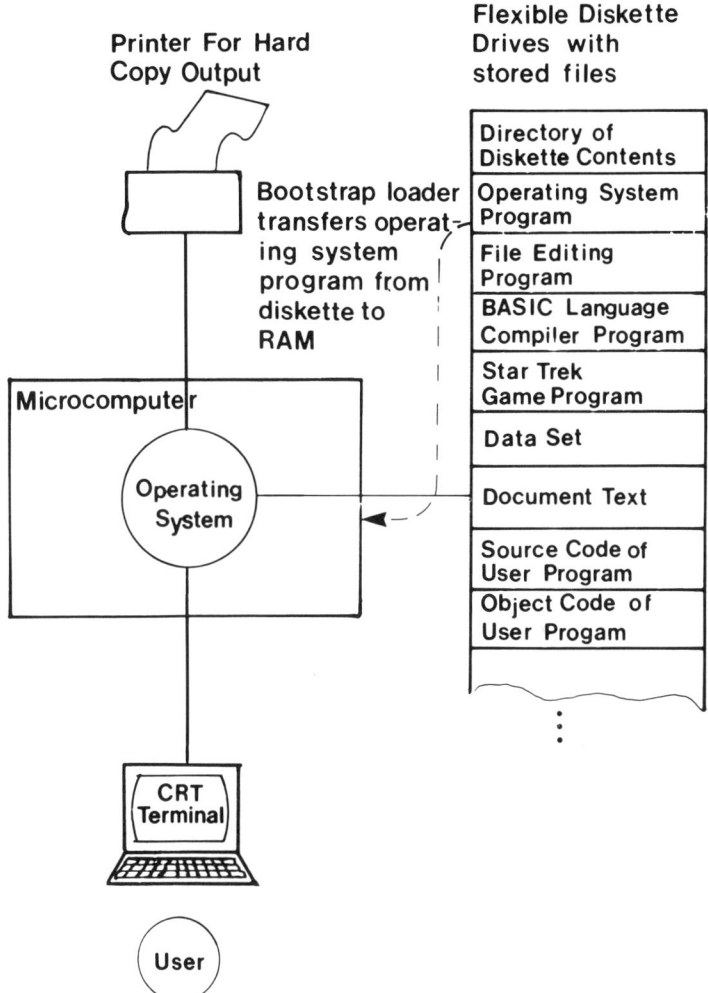

Figure 7. A microcomputer operating system. Initially a bootstrap loader stored in ROM causes the loading into RAM and execution of the operating system program. Then the user, communicating with the system via the CRT terminal, can reach other programs and data stored in files on the flexible diskette.

of a selected portion of a file are displayed on the CRT screen, and the user may enter additions and corrections from the keyboard.

When a file contains a program, the operating system can cause the computer to execute it. Typically a user program is written in one of the many existing computer languages such as FORTRAN (FORmula TRANslator), BASIC (Beginners All-purpose Symbolic Instruction Code) and COBOL (COmmon Business Oriented Language). The text of the program in one of these languages is called the source code. In the first step of execution of the user program, the operating system executes a language translating program called a compiler. The compiler reads the source code file, translates the program into the binary instruction codes used by the CPU, and writes this information, called the object code, into a second file. If the program contains errors, the compiler displays the offending portion of the source code on the CRT along with an error message. The user must then modify the source file using the operating system's editing program to correct the errors and then to compile it again. Such errors are called bugs, and the correction process is termed debugging.* When all the errors have been removed, the operating system can load the object code of the user program into memory and execute it. There is still no guarantee that the program will perform as expected, however. It is very easy to write a program that is syntactically or grammatically correct but which nevertheless does not correctly implement the intended task. The phrase "garbage in, garbage out" (GIGO) has been used to describe this situation.

THE CAPABILITIES AND LIMITATIONS OF COMPUTERS

The capabilities of computers have been outlined in some detail in the preceding sections. They can perform calculations with extreme rapidity; they have enormous memory capacities; they can be made very small and inexpensive; they operate very reliably and accurately; and they can be interfaced easily to control and to monitor processes in the outside world.

The term GIGO mentioned earlier summarizes the limitations of computers in a nutshell. A computer program, regardless of the lan-

---

*When the original ENIAC was constructed, a large number of mechanical relays were included in its architecture. Small insects crawled into the relays, shorting them out and necessitating a process called, appropriately enough, "debugging."

guage in which it is written, must specify a task in terms of input, calculations and comparisons of numbers, storage, and output. This specification, called an algorithm, must be very precise and explicit—all possibilities must be taken into account. It is very easy to write an algorithm to print a table of square roots. It is much more difficult to define an algorithm to control the administration of halothane so that a patient is "appropriately" anesthetized. The key word here is *appropriate*. Unlike computers, anesthesiologists can decide how much halothane is appropriate based on clinical signs, judgment, and experience. If we wish to employ computers in the processes of anesthesia delivery, we must carefully choose the tasks that we will assign to them. It is very difficult to define relatively abstract issues of judgment and experience in the concrete terms of computer algorithms. With this in mind, let us take a look at some of the processes involved in anesthesia delivery with an eye toward possible applications of computers.

PROCESSES OF ANESTHESIA DELIVERY

The goal of anesthesia is rendering a patient insensible to pain, and in the case of general anesthesia, unconscious and immobile as well. These effects on the patient also must be reversible at the conclusion of the surgical procedure. Herein lies the difficulty of anesthesia, because most of the agents we use have narrow margins of safety between their therapeutic and toxic effects. This is particularly true if the patient has several medical illnesses in addition to surgical disease. As anesthesiologists have undertaken the care of sicker patients, more extensive monitoring has become necessary to assure the maintenance of physiologic homeostasis during anesthesia.

As monitoring requirements have become more extensive and as monitoring devices have become more complex, the anesthesiologist has had to devote more attention (sometimes too much attention) to them. Obviously the portion of the anesthesiologist's time that must be devoted to the collection and recording of data from physiologic monitors decreases the amount of time available to interpret the data, to assess the patient clinically, to observe the surgical procedure, to make therapeutic interventions, and to plan the course of the anesthetic. Sometimes there is not enough time left for the latter activities, and the quality of overall anesthetic care is degraded.

If the anesthesiologist does not have enough time to perform adequately all the activities related to anesthesia delivery, then it would be beneficial to have some of these activities handled by other means. One can differentiate the tasks of collection and recording of physiologic data from the other aspects of anesthetic care in that the former are relatively simple and repetitious. They do not require much judgment or experience, and they are disproportionately time-consuming. From the information presented in the preceding sections, it should be clear that these tasks are well suited to handling by computers. Relieved of the tasks of data collection and recording, the anesthesiologist would have much more time available for the overall management of the anesthetic. It should also be clear that the experience, judgment, and skills of the anesthesiologist make the anesthesiologist better suited to this overall management than a computer.

Let us now consider a few of the specific tasks of anesthesia delivery with regard to how computers and anesthesiologists might interact to accomplish them. One of the most important of these is the adequate ventilation and oxygenation of the patient. During anesthesia the patient receives a mixture of oxygen and anesthetic gases through a breathing circuit. Inhalation and exhalation are sometimes spontaneous, but they are usually assisted or controlled by the anesthesiologist by using a handbag or ventilator. Monitoring of oxygenation and ventilation consists usually of sensors of oxygen concentration in the anesthetic circuit, end-tidal carbon dioxide concentration, and airway pressure. During closed-circuit anesthesia, anesthetic circuit volume and patient oxygen consumption are monitored as well.

Arterial blood gas measurements also are obtained when indicated. Many problems can occur with ventilation and oxygenation—a hypoxic gas mixture can be delivered; the breathing circuit or ventilator can malfunction or become disconnected from the patient; the rate of ventilation can be inappropriate; or the patient can develop a pulmonary problem such as bronchospasm or pulmonary edema. Perhaps the most appropriate place for computers initially in this situation would be the continuous monitoring and recording of circuit oxygen concentration, end-tidal carbon dioxide concentration, and airway pressure. The computer could be programmed to warn the anesthesiologist if any of these variables were to fall outside a certain range. This would guard against the delivery of hypoxic gas mixtures and inappropriate rates of ventilation. Failure of the airway pressure to cycle with each breath would indicate a breathing circuit or ventilator malfunction or disconnection. Bronchospasm and pulmonary edema are diagnosed best probably by the anesthesiologist using an esophageal stethoscope.

Another concern of the anesthesiologist is the depth of general anesthesia. This is usually measured by the end-tidal concentration of a volatile or gaseous anesthetic agent, an approximation to the alveolar concentration. Again a computer could be programmed to warn the anesthesiologist if the anesthetic concentration was outside a desired range, and it could record the anesthetic concentration at appropriate intervals. The assessment as to whether a given anesthetic concentration is appropriate for a given patient in a given situation still lies within the domain of the anesthesiologist. Here the use of various clinical signs and past experience play a large role when coupled with close surveillance by the computer.

Muscle relaxation is an important adjunct to many anesthetics. Muscle relaxants are administered intravenously, and their effects are monitored by observation of the mechanical muscle response to stimulation of a peripheral nerve. More recently the electromyographic (EMG) response to stimulation of a peripheral nerve has been used to quantitate the level of muscle relaxation.[4] Although this is primarily a research tool, the potential exists for computer analysis of the EMG signal to produce a digital display of the percentage of neuromuscular blockade in the clinical setting. This could provide a very useful guide to the anesthesiologist in the titration of neuromuscular blocking agents.

The cardiovascular system is perhaps the most extensively monitored physiologic system of the body. The profound effects of anesthetic agents on the cardiovascular system and the life-threatening implications of cardiovascular dysfunction necessitate this. The numerous monitors in common use include the esophageal stethoscope, the electrocardiogram, the plethysmographic pulse transducer, the sphygmomanometer and automatic oscillometric blood pressure measuring device, the intra-arterial cannula, and the flow-directed pulmonary artery thermodilution (Swan-Ganz) catheter. These devices can provide a very large amount of data, especially when a number of them are used simultaneously in a patient with severe cardiovascular disease. Furthermore, there are a number of useful variables such as the rate-pressure product, the tension-time index, and the systemic vascular resistance, to name only a few that can be derived from the data gathered from these monitors. When faced with a severely ill patient experiencing rapid changes in vascular volume and ischemic myocardial dysfunction, the anesthesiologist must be truly agile to collect and to record all the data, to calculate the derived parameters, to interpret the data, and to make the appropriate therapeutic interventions. In this situation, computers could be really useful in collecting data, performing calculations, and displaying data in an organized form to facilitate interpretation by the anesthesiologist. The time thus saved could make the difference between transient myocardial ischemia and an intraoperative myocardial infarction. The computer could also generate an accurate record of events that would otherwise be documented retrospectively and inaccurately in this situation.

Finally, anesthesiologists often monitor various other physiologic variables, such as urine output, body temperature, acid-base balance, and the serum levels of electrolytes and other metabolites. The potential role of computers here would be mainly one of accurate record keeping, although, again, the computer could be programmed to warn the anesthesiologist if a certain parameter was outside its normal range.

It should be emphasized again that at least initially the role of the computer in anesthesia delivery should be to aid in the collection and recording of physiologic data, the calculation of derived variables, and the presentation of the data to the anesthesiologist in an organized, useful form with warnings when parameters lie outside preset limits. This leaves the anesthesiologist with the burdens of data interpretation and therapeutic intervention but allows more time to devote to these tasks.

Assuming the successful integration of computers into the practice of anesthesiology as data gatherers and recorders, the question arises as to the next step. The answer is clearly in the direction of automatic control. For example, one could program a computer-controlled ventilator to maintain a desired end-tidal carbon dioxide concentration by automatically adjusting the ventilatory frequency and tidal volume. One could also program a computer-controlled infusion pump to administer neuromuscular blocking agents to maintain a desired level of neuromuscular blockade based on EMG measurements. Indeed, an infusion system that administers sodium nitroprusside to maintain desired mean arterial pressure has been in everyday clinical use for several years.[5] These automatic control systems must be implemented with great care, however. The anesthesiologist still must be warned when abnormal situations develop; the equipment must be able to detect malfunctions of its components; and there must be built-in fail-safe devices and manual backup capabilities. If implemented in this manner, automatic control systems have the potential to free even more of the anesthesiologist's time for other tasks of anesthetic management. Thus the patient should receive safer anesthesia.

DO WE NEED COMPUTERS NOW?

Many would argue that computers are unnecessary because anesthesiologists have successfully practiced their art without the encumbrance of computer technology since W.T.G. Morton first administered ether in 1846, a century before the construction of the ENIAC. This is difficult to refute for two reasons. First, most patients undergoing anesthesia are reasonably healthy. These patients tolerate wide variations in anesthetic technique and even many errors in anesthetic management without suffering any irreversible harm. Secondly, most problems that occur during anesthesia can be handled sucessfully by the judgment and skill of experienced anesthesiologists before any harm comes to the patient. This is the basis of the "art" of anesthesia, and many would argue that computers and art are not compatible.

But there are others who believe that anesthesiology should be a quantitative science as well as an art. The basis of science is the collection of objective data and the formulation of decisions based on this data and a set of rules or decision tree. There is no question that computers can be appropriately applied to the collection of objective data; indeed, this process has already begun. The real challenge facing anesthesiologists in the next several years is the critical examination of what we call "judgment and experience" leading to the formation of decision-making rules (algorithms) to use with the data that we will have in abundance. When we have developed these algorithms, computers will be even more useful and probably necessary for their practical implementation.

We need computers now; without the aid of these powerful tools, we cannot develop the full potential of the science of anesthesiology.

REFERENCES

1. GOLDSTINE, HH: *The Computer from Pascal to von Neumann.* Princeton University Press, Princeton, 1972, pp 157–166.
2. LEVINE, RD: *Supercomputers.* Sci Am 246(1):118–135, January, 1982.
3. BURKS, AW, GOLDSTINE, HH, VON NEUMANN, JL: *Preliminary discussion of the logical design of an electronic computing instrument.* Princeton, June 28, 1946. Reprinted in BELL, CG, NEWELL, A: *Computer Structures: Readings and Examples.* McGraw-Hill, New York, 1971.

4. RITCHIE, RG: A system for the automatic control of muscle relaxation in surgical patients. Unpublished data.
5. SHEPPARD, LC: *Computer control of the infusion of vasoactive drugs.* Ann Biomed Eng 8:431–444, 1980.

BIBLIOGRAPHY

Byte Magazine. Published monthly by Byte Publications, Peterborough, New Hampshire.

GOLDSTEIN, HH: *The Computer from Pascal to von Neumann.* Princeton University Press, Princeton, 1972.

MEINDL, JD: *Microelectronics and computers in medicine.* Science 215(4534):792–797, February 12, 1982.

PORTER, K: *Computers Made Really Simple.* Crowell, New York, 1976.

SLOTNICK, DL AND SLOTNICK, JK: *Computers: Their Structure, Use, and Influence.* Prentice-Hall, Englewood Cliffs, 1979.

VANDAM, LD: *Simplicity and common sense in anesthesia.* Med Instrum 14(3):157–159, May–June, 1980.

WEIZENBAUM, J: *Computer Power and Human Reason from Judgment to Calculation.* WH Freeman, San Francisco, 1976.

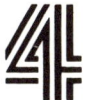

STANDARDS FOR ANESTHESIA: THE ISSUES
Leslie Rendell-Baker, M.D.

THE ASA AND THE ANSI Z79 STANDARDS COMMITTEE

Who Needs Standards?

"Why does our society have to support a standards committee? Why don't the manufacturers write the standards? And what use are standards in my practice anyway?"

I am sure many anesthesiologists have from time to time questioned the value of their society's long-continued support of standards activities which appear to produce no immediate results. However, if one wants a true estimate of improvement produced by this work it is only necessary to reflect why the multiple mask adapter (Fig. 1) introduced in 1949 was such a great breakthrough.[1] It enabled one to use any make of mask with any make of breathing system! Today that is no big deal, for we take for granted that any mask will fit any breathing system; but in 1949 each make of machine had its own size of breathing attachments, so that only Foregger breathing attachments would fit the Foregger machine. The same applied for Ohio, McKesson, and all the others. The plight of anesthesiologists before the introduction of the standard 22- and 15-mm sizes was somewhat similar to that of the international traveler who wishes to use an electrical appliance in each country visited. Merely to plug it into the local electrical outlets

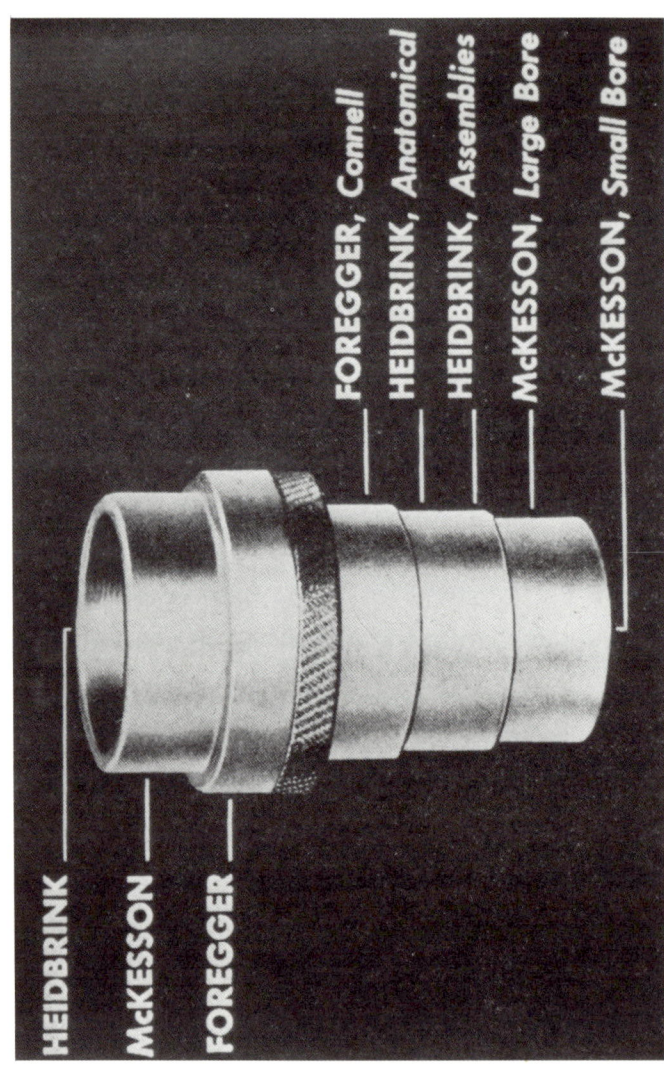

Figure 1. Weiss' Universal Mask Adapter (1949). In 1949, before the adoption of the standard 22 mm fitting for the breathing system, this was a most useful device because it permitted the use of eight different combinations of three different sizes of mask adapters and masks with five different sizes and genders of mask orifices.

in foreign countries, the traveler is likely to need the selection of multiple adapters shown in Figure 2.

The American Society of Anesthetists (as it was then called) had a standardization committee working on these problems before World War II. The practical difficulties they faced were vividly recounted by Ralph Tovell,[2] who reported that in 1942 the US Army in Britain was using four makes of anesthesia apparatus, each of which took a different size expendable part, so that one could never be sure in an emergency which type of equipment would fit the machine in use.

In 1955, the ASA Committee on Standards took the initiative. In 1956, the American National Standards Committee Z79 on Anesthesia and Respiratory Equipment was formed. It was our ASA colleagues' tenacity and determination that has made a success of national and international standards for anesthesia equipment.

Hamilton S. Davis, M.D., of Cleveland, then chairman of Z79, approached Congresswoman Frances Payne Bolton for assistance in sending a delegation to the first US/UK joint anesthesia standards meeting in London in July, 1959. The congresswoman asked a knowledgeable physician in the defense department for an opinion on the merit of the project. He replied that it was a hopeless cause, for how could these anesthesiologists obtain the agreement of US and UK manufacturers and physicians, when he could not even get agreement between the US Army and Navy on standard medical equipment? In spite of this depressing advice, Congresswoman Bolton financed our flight to Britain, and through our department chairman, Bob Hingson, (whose brother was in the US Navy) we were able to arrange for the US Navy to bring us back aboard the aircraft carrier USS Lake Champlain when it called in Edinburgh before returning to the USA at the end of that summer's naval exercises.

Needless to say, we were determined to prove the defense department's doomsayer wrong. However, he was accurate in saying that the task was not easy, and certainly initial progress was far from rapid.

Agreement on the method of sizing of tracheal tubes by the internal diameter in millimeters instead of the arbitrary Magill numbers (from 00 to 10) or the French system of numbers (the circumference or outside diameter $\times$ 3) was achieved at that July, 1958, meeting. The US members also brought back for study the proposed British standard anesthesia breathing systems using size 23 mm conical fittings. US/UK agreement to adopt the 22 mm diameter fitting was achieved in December, 1958. This was followed in December, 1959, by the adoption of the 15 mm male and female fittings previously used for

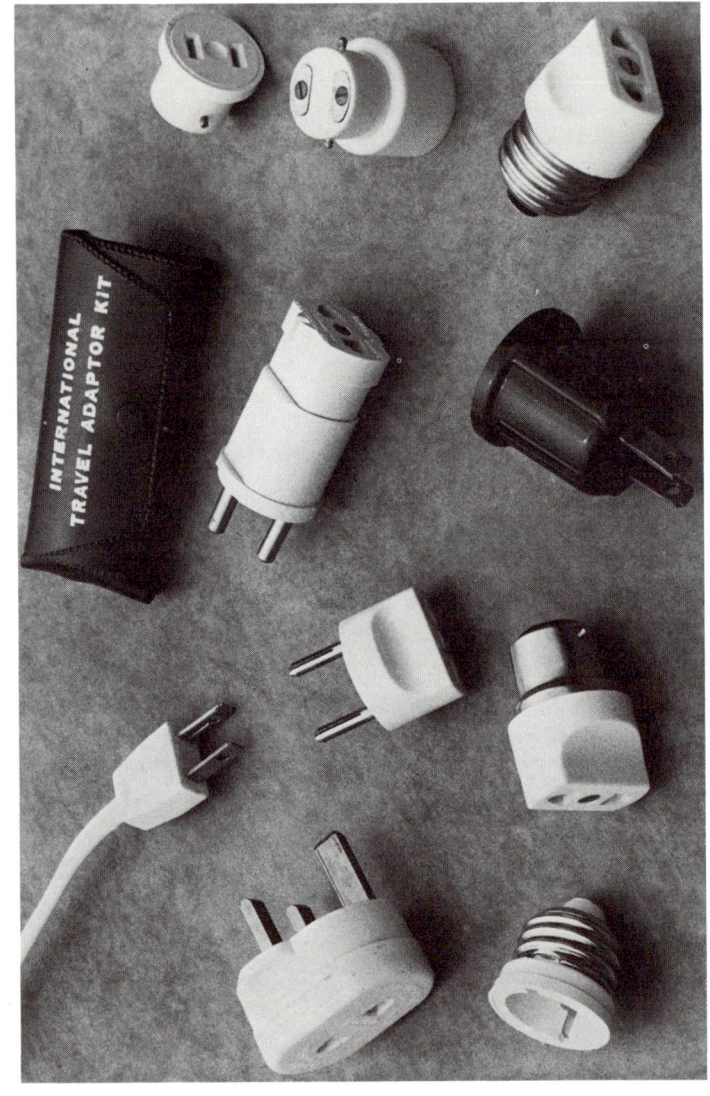

Figure 2. The US Plug Meets Its European Relatives! No single standard for electrical outlets in Europe makes these adapters essential for the international traveler.

endotracheal tube connectors for use in the pediatric breathing system. The precise design of the gauges to check the accuracy of the male and female 15 mm and 22 mm breathing fitting were hammered out at a meeting in London in June, 1964, and the British standard based on this agreement was published in 1965.[3] This has now been incorporated into a draft international standard (ISO/D1S5356/1 and 2), which we hope will be adopted in 1983 and will be followed by the publication of the US equivalent standard.

At the urging of Ralph Tovell, the adult 22 mm size orifice was adopted for pediatric face masks, so that in an emergency, anes-

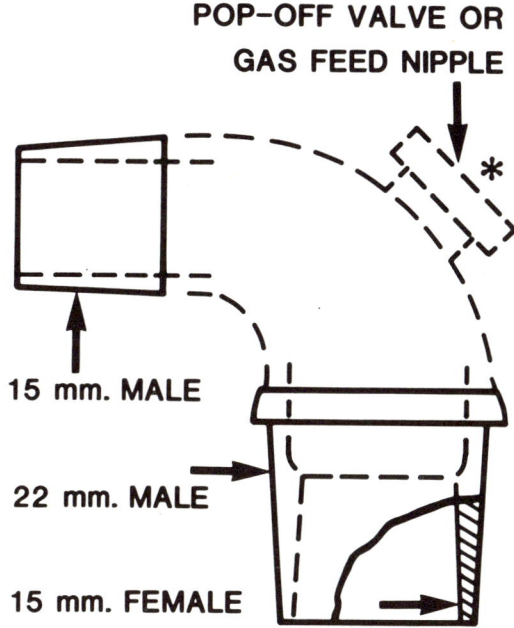

PEDIATRIC MASK ADAPTER

Figure 3. Pediatric Mask Adapter 1961. This original drawing from the 1961 draft standard of the pediatric breathing system indicated by the dotted line that the precise design, apart from the 15 mm and 22 mm connections, could be varied to meet individual requirements. A version without the pop-off valve or gas feed nipple forms a part of most present-day breathing systems. (From *Problems with Anesthetic and Respiratory Therapy Equipment.* Int Anesthesiol Clin 20 (3): 177, 1982, with permission.)

thesia could be conducted using a pediatric face mask with adult size equipment. Because the rest of the pediatric equipment had 15 mm size fittings, it was necessary to evolve a 22 mm to 15 mm mask adapter for the pediatric system. This adapter was given a 15 mm internal diameter so that it could connect either a tracheal tube or face mask to the breathing system (Fig. 3). This mask adapter was also found extremely convenient for adults and has long since become a standard piece of equipment in all disposable and reusable anesthesia breathing systems. Pediatric circle absorption systems such as the Bloomquist (formerly widely used) have become less popular. Thus for children between 12 and 20 kg, the adult circle absorption system is commonly used with less compliant, smaller tubing which has less internal compressible volume.

None of this disposable breathing equipment could have been developed if standard-sized fittings were not used on all our anesthesia breathing equipment. It would not be economically possible for a manufacturer to make four or five different-size breathing systems and sell them as disposable. It is only by the use of standard sizes and fittings that the necessary volume and economy can be made which permits the development of a disposable equipment industry whose turnover this year is estimated to be $100 million.

EXAMPLES OF STANDARDIZATION

22 mm and 15 mm Fittings

Originally both male and female 22 mm and 15 mm fittings were made of metal. However, now almost all the female fittings are made of flexible plastic, rubber, or other elastomeric materials. The male fittings, too, are often made of plastic.

These fittings, when made of metal to the standard dimensions, provided a secure fit that was unlikely to become disengaged accidentally. However, though it may be relatively easy to maintain accuracy in metal parts, when the same parts are made of plastic, shrinkage and distortion may occur. As a result, many plastic components[4,5] have been shown to diverge widely from the standard shape and sizes. Accidental disconnection of the patient from the breathing system between the tracheal tube connector and Y piece has unfortunately become all too common.

An essential first step toward solving this problem is to modify the molds so that the plastic fittings produced will satisfy the standard gauge tests. The ANSI MD 70 committee, which is working on a revision of the 1955 standard for Luer Taper fittings, has solved this problem of the change from rigid materials (metal, glass) to plastic by insisting upon the use of accurate plug and ring gauges for testing all components. The 6 percent conical tapered shape and dimensional tolerances of the female fitting are maintained the same, regardless of materials. However, though a plastic male fitting is made with the same conical taper, it can be made slightly larger in diameter to allow for the plastic component's tendency to give when firmly engaged with the opposite component.

This committee has evolved an anti-disengagement performance test[6] in which the component is assembled to the test piece with a force of 25N (5.5 lb) followed by an attempted 45° axial rotation. The same force of 25N but without rotation is then applied gradually in the opposite direction, maintained for 10 seconds and then quickly released. The fitting shall remain attached to the test fixture. Such a test no doubt could also be used to evaluate the surface characteristics of plastic breathing system fittings, some of which have a high coefficient of retention, but others have all the retentive characteristics of candle wax or a bar of soap!

To limit the amount of distortion owing to shrinkage, some manufacturers have reduced the thickness of the plastic by incorporating multiple grooves in the 22 mm male mask adapter. The draft ISO and US standards on breathing system fittings incorporated such grooves in the mask adapter at the request of the German Drager Company, who asserted that the grooves provided a more secure fit in the face mask. There would be no functional harm in incorporating such grooves in other conical fittings, if desired.

Adult Breathing Circuit Layout

The original US/UK breathing systems of 1965 incorporated a "gas flow sequence" of male-female fittings to deal with the potential hazard of two sets of unidirectional valves (one in the Y piece and the other on the absorber) being accidentally incorporated in a breathing system in opposition. This would prevent the patient from being ventilated. The British-made hard-rubber male and female fittings used by many US manufacturers for the 1967 field trials of these circuits unfortunately distorted, particularly when autoclaved. Thus, they no longer provided a secure fit and fell apart in use. As a result, the adult "gas flow sequence" breathing system was withdrawn in the US, pending further work and trials at the international level.

This produced Draft International Standard 5356/1 and 2, which is expected to be adopted in a formal vote in 1983. The circle system in this draft standard is the simple layout that has come into general use in the US. It is identical to that proposed by the British committee in July, 1958, except that the British system used 23 mm fittings.

In the absence of any active consideration of an American National Standard on breathing system fittings after 1965, the Compressed Gas Association in 1972 published in their pamphlet *M1 Standard for 22 mm Anesthesia Circuit Connectors* the precise dimensions of the 22 mm fittings and the 15/22 mm mask fittings for the guidance of designers. These fittings had by then been widely incorporated into most manufacturers' designs.

More recently, problems have arisen when new young designers, coming into the standards field and viewing the wide variability of the actual dimensions of plastic components, have concluded that there were no standard dimensions for 15 mm and 22 mm fittings. This error particularly applied to manufacturers of ventilators, because the 1976 American standard on breathing machines for medical use did not illustrate these fittings but merely referred to them in other standards documents. As a result, a few manufacturers have used 22 mm diameter male fittings but have ignored the standard 1 in 40 taper. Though this deviation from the standard may not appear significant when these fittings mate only with female elastomeric components, the use of such nonstandard fittings does make it impossible to attach other devices to the ventilator except by using short lengths of rubber hose. This is also the case with many humidifiers, which as a result cannot be attached directly to anesthesia apparatus.

Puritan-Bennett has evolved for their ventilator a disposable breathing system that incorporates special antidisconnect fittings approximately 22 mm in diameter. These fittings accept only their specially designed disposable hoses. Although this system may provide a significant improvement, it locks the user into one manufacturer for supply of disposable breathing systems.

It was precisely to avoid this situation that the Z79 standards committee started in 1956. If this trend spreads and each manufacturer produces its own specific circuit, we will soon be back where we started with 10 ventilators and 10 breathing systems—none of which is interchangeable or compatible.

Manufacturers have complained that though the 1 in 40 male conical fitting might be satisfactory for metal to metal fittings, they do not provide the best purchase for an elastomeric hose or reservoir bag.

As a result of user complaints, Ohio Medical Products have reverted to their earlier cylindrical bag mount with an expanded olive tip over which the neck of the bag must be forced. The use of such a nonstandard fitting for the bag mount may not pose a significant problem, provided all manufacturers make their bag mount fittings of the same diameter with the same size of expansion at the mouth of the fitting.

Standards for Ventilators

A standard for ventilators evolved under the chairmanship of the late Dr. Meyer Saklad and was published in 1976. For the first time, this provided a standard series of resistances and compliances against which ventilators could be tested. Since 1976, many different functions have been added to the ventilator, necessitating an expansion of the test methods and test apparatus. An updated standard should be available in the near future.

Standard on Performance of Anesthesia Breathing Systems

Dr. Meyer Saklad did such an excellent job in evolving the test parameters for the ventilator standard that when similar features were needed for the performance of anesthesia breathing systems he was the unanimous choice for the task. With the benefit of an FDA contract, his laboratory tested and delineated the performance to be expected from all components of breathing systems. The proposed standard on the performance and safety requirements for anesthesia breathing systems, now awaiting ballot, is based largely on Meyer Saklad and colleagues' work.

The need to add humidity to the gases in the circle absorption system both to maintain the patient's temperature and to prevent damage to the bronchial mucosa has been brought to our attention by the work of Chalon and colleagues.[7]

Anesthesiologists, unlike respiratory therapists, tend to be unmindful of the amount of the anesthesia ventilator's tidal volume, which is lost into the compliant breathing tubes and the system's considerable internal compressible volume. On one typical system, 360 ml of gas was "lost" at 30 cm water pressure.

Coté and colleagues have shown that the trend in anesthesia for pediatric patients to use a combination of a heated humidifier, an adult circle absorber, compliant breathing tubing, and controlled ventilation has highlighted the importance of system compliance.[8]

When a system pressure of 40 cm water was needed to ventilate the patient, with some systems no gas would be delivered to the patient. For these patients a Mapleson D system with noncompliant tubing gave better results.

STANDARDS REQUIRED FOR THE FUTURE

Standards To Prevent Disconnections

There is no doubt that the most urgent problem facing clinicians and manufacturers on anesthesia standards committees is the problem of accidental disconnection of the patient from the breathing system during anesthesia and ventilatory care. As a temporary solution, hooks, knobs, and other protuberances were added by manufacturers to Y pieces and elbow connections to permit the use of elastic bands and other means to prevent accidental separation of the components.

Anesthesiologists have been unable to agree on how securely the tube connector, Y piece, and other breathing system components should be connected together. The fear is that the hazard of accidental disconnection will be exchanged for the even greater hazard of accidental extubation of the patient's trachea. A study is now underway, funded by the US Food and Drug Administration (FDA) and the Canadian Health Protection Branch of the Canadian Health and Welfare Department, to ascertain the incidence of accidental disconnection and to recommend the most satisfactory solutions to the problem.

Standards for Transcutaneous Oxygen Monitors

Though a considerable amount of work on the use of transcutaneous oxygen monitors has been done, particularly in children, the results obtained in adults have been highly variable. A Z79 subcommittee is studying the problem, and it is hoped that a standard on the performance and testing of these devices may help.

HUMAN ENGINEERING OF MEDICAL DEVICES

During the work that resulted in the publication of the Z79.8 standard on the performance and safety on anesthesia gas machines, it became clear that many of the hazards were due to the poor human engineering of the apparatus. This problem also extended to many medical devices. For this reason, guidelines on the human engineering of medical devices have been produced by a committee of the Association for Advancement of Medical Instrumentation (AAMI).

It is likely that future revisions of Z79.8 will lay even greater emphasis on the needs for careful integration of the design of anesthesia apparatus incorporating good human engineering principles, so that the apparatus will be simple, straightforward, and unconfusing to the user.

Within the next decade, the electronic revolution that has swept through the laboratory and industry should lead to anesthesia apparatus that monitor their own functions and those of the user. It is clear from the ready acceptance of the Dinamap (Critikon) and other automatic blood pressure recording devices that anesthesiologists would welcome equipment that would take care of the simple repetitive recording and charting that occupies so much time during anesthesia.

The primary advantages of such devices are demonstrated during induction and moments of crisis when much of the anesthesiologist's attention must be devoted to urgent restorative measures. Automatic recording devices could document clearly what transpired rather than the anesthesiologist being left, as at present, to reconstruct what happened, as best can be determined, when stability has been restored.

A committee of AAMI has produced a draft standard on automatic blood pressure recording devices. This draft should be a helpful first step toward a uniform standard of function and safety for this new equipment.

ALARM STANDARDS: HYPOXIC ACCIDENTS

Failure To Use the Oxygen Analyzer

Hypoxic accidents during anesthesia continue to occur even though oxygen analyzers are available.[9] Anesthesiologists either forget or neglect to turn on the device routinely before the start of anesthesia. Hospital authorities responsible for minimizing the impact of malpractice claims on their hospitals have expressed a strong desire that the activation of oxygen analyzers should be made automatic so that the analyzer will function whenever gases are flowing from the machine, as on the North American Drager Model Narkomed 2A. It may be some time before the US national standard Z79.10 can reflect such a requirement. It is more likely that the purchasing power of such concerned hospital authorities will bring forth such a device.

Disconnection Alarms

Accidental disconnection of the apneic patient from the anesthesia breathing system while the ventilation is being provided by a volume ventilator is an all too frequent occurrence. Unfortunately, some of the alarms that have been available have failed to signal when disconnection occurred.[9,10,11] Alarms in the future should be designed to recognize the normal breathing pattern and should alarm if significant change in it occurs.[12]

Accidental Pulmonary Barotrauma

A problem in the reverse direction has been the accidental exposure of the patient's lungs to high pressure.[13] Excessive pressure can arise in several ways: 1) from accidental activation of the oxygen flush,[14] which may rupture the lungs before the patient can be disconnected from the system; 2) from a prolonged period of increasing pressure

Table 1. Recommended Features for Pressure Alarm Safety Mechanisms

1. It should detect the loss of normal pressure fluctuations in the breathing system and sound an alarm.
2. Flow of gases should be monitored simultaneously with pressure variations, so that spontaneous versus mandatory ventilation can be detected. If no flow occurs, or if a spontaneous flow pattern is detected while the ventilation mode is on, an alarm should sound.
3. If the pressure in the breathing system exceeds 30 cm H_2O for too long (e.g., 5 sec), the device should release the pressure and sound the alarm. After the breathing system pressure has been at atmospheric pressure for 5 seconds, the mechanism could close the system again and allow the pressure to increase to 30 cm H_2O before opening once more. This would provide artificial respiration while sounding the alarm.
4. Should the pressure in the breathing system ever exceed a dangerous transient pressure (e.g., 50 cm H_2O), the mechanism should open the system and sound the alarm. Again, after a 5-second pause at atmospheric pressure, the valve should close and open once again when the pressure reaches 30 cm H_2O. By repeating the cycle, artificial respiration can be provided as the alarm is sounding until reset by the operator.
5. Activation of the high-pressure alarm and pressure-relief mechanism should be automatic with the switching on of the flow of anesthesia gases. The mechanism should be incorporated into or attached to the anesthesia apparatus. The disconnect alarm should become operative automatically with switching on of the anesthesia ventilator.

from incorrect connection of the patient to a ventilator;[15] 3) from failure to adjust properly the pressure relief valve;[16] and 4) from faulty scavenging systems.

Though the latest model of the North American Drager DPM-S pressure monitor responds to these situations, it is desirable that in addition to sounding an alarm the apparatus should promptly release the pressure from the breathing system. However, should the breathing system then remain open, an apneic patient could become anoxic unless an alert attendant responds quickly to the emergency. The invaluable features of a combined alarm-safety mechanism have been recommended and are summarized in Table 1.[13]

INFLUENCE OF FDA BUREAU OF MEDICAL DEVICES ON STANDARDS

When medical devices legislation was first proposed, the initial response of the FDA staff who handled approval of new drugs was that they would process a new device in the same way. To anesthesiologists and manufacturers, this meant "very slowly," so both opposed early medical devices legislation.

However, industry eventually concluded that some medical device legislation was inevitable. Manufacturers and clinicians then worked through AAMI and other organizations for the adoption of legislation more reasonable than that applicable to drugs.

The presence of staff of the Bureau of Medical Devices as members of standards committees has signified the bureau's commitment to handling a significant part of device control through standards achieved by voluntary consensus. Previously, participants less than 100 percent committed to the objectives of a standards committee's work might try to be obstructive. This is no longer a reasonable attitude when it is clear that the majority on the committee consider the requirements and tests in question to be acceptable.

The bureau made a permanent change in the standards being written by insisting that there be a Rationale and Referee Test Method for every requirement in the standard. ANSI and ISO had never included these in their standards but have done so since ANSI Z79.8, the standard on gas machine performance and safety.

Performance Standards

The emphasis of the medical device legislation on performance standards, which has been stressed by the FDA's participants in standards writing, has led some people to feel erroneously that performance standards are all that are needed. Imagine what the US would be like without the standard two-bladed electrical plug, with each state using a different plug.

The standard connections between apparatus such as the Luer fittings used for intravenous equipment and the 15 and 22 mm connections used in anesthesia form the very backbone of a system. Without the standard connection, nothing will work. No amount of performance standards will help.

Color Standards

STANDARD COLORS FOR VOLATILE ANESTHETIC CONTAINERS

When the Canadian standard on the agent-specific vaporizer filling system was published, it incorporated a keyed flexible plastic filler which connected the bottle to the vaporizer.[17] The necks of the bottles were of differing size, and the filler for each agent had a specific color: red for halothane, orange for enflurane, and so forth. A keyed plastic collar was added to the bottle of volatile agent. This, too, was the same color as the filler.

When the patent on halothane expired, several companies entered the market. One of them used a label on their bottle with an orange

Table 2. Recommended Colors for Volatile Anesthetic Agent Container Labels and Agent Specific Filling System

Drug	Color	Federal (#594a) standard color	British BS5252 color	Pantone (21)	Munsell*
Halothane	Red	11105	04 E 56	200	5R 4/14
Enflurane	Orange	22510	06 E 55	144	2.5YR 6/16
Methoxyflurane	Green	14187	14 E 53	334	10G 5/10
Trichlorethylene†	Blue	15102	20 E 56	294	2.5PB3/8
Spare	Yellow	13655	10 E 55	116	3.75Y 8/14
Spare	Gray	16251	00 A 09	430	5PB 5/1
Isoflurane	Purple	None		252/253	10P 4/12

*Munsell color for Isoflurane confirmed May 28, 1980.
†No longer available in USA.

If the manufacturer wishes to use color on any of the above items, then these are the ones recommended. A black-and-white label may also be used for any agent.
From Table I in ISO/TC 121/SC1 (UK) N300 July 1980

panel very similar in shape and color to that used on the enflurane bottle. This ill-advised action was followed by a report[18] of an accidental filling of a keyed enflurane vaporizer with halothane from a bottle with the orange label and without a collar. The anesthesiologist had managed to force the keyed filling adapter onto the halothane bottle well enough to fill the enflurane vaporizer. Following this, the tolerances on the flexible plastic fillers were tightened and a proposed international agreement on the colors to be used with the volatile agents was achieved (Table 2). In the future only these colors, or black and white, should be used to label the box and bottle of the agent, the plastic filler and collar, and the vaporizer itself.

A much improved vaporizer keyed filling mechanism has been developed which fills much faster and uses only one orifice for both filling and emptying. The international standard incorporating this filling mechanism and the standard range of colors should be ready for approval within the next year or so.

STANDARD COLORS FOR ANESTHESIA SYRINGE LABELS

Prior to inducing anesthesia with fentanyl-thiopental-succinylcholine, a colleague had filled and labeled two 5 ml syringes, one with fentanyl and the other with succinylcholine. As was his practice, he injected a preliminary dose of fentanyl before giving the thiopental. He was horrified to see that his patient, instead of becoming drowsy, grimaced as he became paralyzed from the mistaken injection of succinylcholine. This was an experience both patient and anesthesiologist would rather not remember. Later examination of the syringe labels showed that newly acquired labels had very similar colors for both fentanyl and succinylcholine. The colors of the previously used labels had been quite different.

This colleague's problem was not unique, as the following extract from a letter indicates:

> I received your information on your anesthetic labels. I think your label system is terrible. I can't see how your company would decide to market labels for different drugs with the same color code and for the same drug with different colors. For example, same drug: Pentothal-blue and sodium pentothal-aqua, Anectine-white, succinylcholine-lavender. Different drugs: Arfonad, Curare, Lidocaine and Valium-red. I would think that you would do more study of the market before you expose yourself and the product to possible liability action. (J.S.I., personal communication.)

Table 3. Proposed Standard Colors for Drug Syringe Labels*

Drug class	Examples	Pantone color (all uncoated)
1 Induction agents	Thiopental, methohexital thiamylal, diazepam	Yellow
2 Anesthetic agents	Ketamine	Violet 251
3 Muscle relaxants	Succinylcholine,* Curare, metocurine, gallamine pancuronium, epicuronium, atracuronium	Red 185
3a Relaxant antagonists	Neostigimine, endrophonium pyridostigmine	Red 185 and white diagonal stripes
4 Narcotics	Morphine, fentanyl, meperidine	Blue 297
4a Narcotic antagonists	Levallorphan, naloxone	Blue 297 and white diagonal stripes
5 Major tranquilizers	Droperidol, chlorpromazine	Brown 470
5b Combination of narcotics and major tranquilizers	Innovar, fentanyl-droperidol combination	Blue 297 and brown 470 longitudinal stripes
6 Vasopressors	Epinephrine,* ephedrine neosynephrine	Orange 151
6a Hypotensive agents	Trimetaphan, nitroprusside, nitroglycerine, phentolamine	Orange 151 and white diagonal stripes
7 Local anesthetics	Procaine, lidocaine	Gray 402
8 Anticholinergic agents	Atropine, glycopyrrolate	Green 367

*Color coding of the background of the label or tape applied to the syringe is suggested. All printing is to be a minimum of 20 point (with letters 5 mm high) in black bold type, with the exception that the words succinylcholine and epinephrine should be printed in white type. The examples shown are representative, not restrictive.

All other drugs should be labeled with black printing on white background.

One cannot argue with the latter opinion, but a printer wishing to enter this market at present would have difficulty in obtaining reliable advice on which colors to use for which drugs. For if one works in several hospitals, the possibility for confusion is ever present, because each label company has its own ideas of a color code.

With the benefit of hindsight, it is clear that a uniform code would be helpful. In this country, Turndorf and Wang have advocated this, and the South African Society of Anaesthetists' Standards Committee[19] and the British Medico-Pharmaceutical Forum[20] investigating dangerous mistakes in drug administration have also explored the idea. The American Society of Testing and Materials D10.34 subcommittee proposed a color code for anesthesia syringe labels, based on the South African proposals.

Rather than relying upon names for the colors to be used, the precise number in the Pantone color code[21] used by printers should be given (Table 3). The colors distinguish the groups from each other with clear bold lettering used to identify the specific members of a group. Thus, all relaxants will have the same red label with the name **CURARE, PANCURONIUM,** and so forth printed in black. To distinguish it from the other relaxants it is proposed that **SUCCINYLCHOLINE** be printed in white on a red label. Definite saturated colors have been chosen rather than pastel shades to minimize the problems of 8 percent males with errors in color vision.

Standards for Pharmaceuticals

LABELS FOR AMPULES AND SMALL-VOLUME CONTAINERS OF PHARMACEUTICALS

Although nongaseous drugs seem to have little to do with anesthesia delivery systems, unambiguous identification and correct dosage are amenable to systematic control, as is record keeping. The misreading and misidentification of ampules and other drug containers is a problem which has bedeviled all branches of medicine and nursing. Interest developed by Dr. Wang and Dr. Turndorf with their graphic demonstration of the similarity of the container and label for drugs of widely dissimilar action led to the formation of the American Society of Testing and Materials subcommittee D10.34.* This subcommittee has issued a draft standard intended to ensure that the label is at least legible.

---

*Another subcommittee of the D10 committee evolved the child-proof closures for drug containers.

Smellie, Lees, and Smith studied how nurses and anesthetists located a drug container in order to read the label.[22] This is important because before the label can be read, the container must first be located. Nurses found the expected location of the container in the medication cart followed by the size of the container to be most useful. Anesthesiologists placed the color, followed by the distinctive shape of the container, as most useful features in locating the correct drug.

Nurses rigorously trained to read the label always did so. To help them, they suggested that drugs be stored in single rows, so that clear informative labels could be read without lifting the containers. This would require large bold lettering for legibility. The anesthetist's use of color and distinctive shape of containers could be exploited by introducing color coding of groups of similar drugs, i.e., hypnotics, analgesics, muscle relaxants, vasopressors, and so forth. They recommended that drugs liable to be confused be bought from manufacturers using widely different shaped containers.

I have no doubt that the alternative, standard container shapes would meet with manufacturers' resistance. For example, Burroughs Wellcome would be unhappy if all firms supplied succinylcholine in 30 ml rectangular bottles similar to theirs, but this, according to Smellie, Lees, and Smith's study, would greatly enhance correct recognition of the drug.

ASTM Subcommittee D10.34 may follow this British study by exploring the use of their color code for syringe labels on the labels for ampules and vials of the same drugs. Later, possibly, shapes of drug containers could be considered.

DRUGS SUPPLIED IN SYRINGES FOR IMMEDIATE INJECTION

Manufacturers have made available drugs commonly used in emergency situations that are packaged in syringes ready for immediate injection. One of these drugs is lidocaine in 2 percent solution (100 mg in 5 ml). The bolus dose of lidocaine is commonly followed by an infusion of dilute lidocaine (0.2 percent). In addition, manufacturers have also provided syringes with 1 and 2 grams of 20 percent solution that are readily available for immediate injection into a bottle of intravenous fluid in order to prepare the dilute solution.

Unfortunately, in the heat of the moment, there have been numerous occasions reported when staff in the intensive care unit or emergency room injected the 20 percent solution rather than the 2 percent solution into the patient, with lethal results. Many hospitals have refused to stock the 20 percent solution of lidocaine in syringes.

Unfortunately, once removed from their prominently labeled and colored boxes, these syringes are often similar in appearance to other syringes. As a result, there have been reports of epinephrine being administered instead of lidocaine[23] and of bupivacaine being given instead of sodium bicarbonate.[24]

It would seem reasonable that only drugs to be injected in an emergency be placed in such syringes. Drugs that are intended to be diluted before being given intravenously should not be supplied in a container that would permit their being injected either into an IV injection port or directly into a patient's vein. Not only should it not be possible to make such an injection, but it is desirable that the container does not resemble a syringe, for if it does some ingenious person will certainly make an intravenous injection with it.

Narcotics and sedative drugs such as morphine, meperidine, and diazepam are commonly supplied in small syringes or Tubex components ready for injection. These are not a problem, for it is highly unlikely that the wrong drug will be withdrawn from the drug cabinet and entered into the control register. This is a deliberate process requiring the identification of the drug, recording of the patient's name with dose, and the number of units remaining in stock. In any case, it is unlikely that the administration of a larger than intended dose of these controlled drugs intravenously would have catastrophic effects.

It is to be hoped that the ASTM D10.34 subcommittee will be able to evolve a safe code of practice for drugs to be marketed in preloaded syringes ready for use. (An alternative method requiring more technologic support would involve bar coding of prefilled syringes with a light pen or similar device connected to an inexpensive microprocessor-controlled data system with all the commonly marketed drugs in its memory for final check prior to administration.—*Ed.*)

REFERENCES

1. WEISS, WA: *Universal mask adapter.* Anesthesiology 10:233–234, 1949.
2. TOVELL, RM: *Problems in supply of anesthetic gases in the European theater of operations.* U.S. Army. Anesthesiology 8:303–311, 1947.
3. British Standard 3849:1965 Breathing Attachments for Anaesthetic Apparatus.
4. SHAW, A, DAVIS, PD, ANDERSON, IM: *Tapered connectors in patient breathing systems.* Anaesthesia 37:201–203, 1982.
5. NEUFELD, PD, SINCLAIR, AS, JOHNSON, DL: *Anti-disconnect strategies for anaesthesia breathing circuits.* From Bureau of Medical Devices,

National Health and Welfare, Canada AAMI 17th Annual Meeting Abstracts, May, 1982.
6. ANSI MD 70.1-1982 Performance Standard for Medical Luer Taper Fittings.
7. CHALON, J, ET AL: *Humidification of Anesthetic Gases.* Thomas, Springfield. 1981.
8. COTÉ, CJ, ET AL: *Wasted ventilation with eight anesthetic circuits used on children.* Anesthesiology 55:A334, September, 1981.
9. RENDELL-BAKER, L AND MEYER, JA: *Failure to use O_2 analyzers to prevent hypoxic accidents.* Anesthesiology 58:287-288, 1983.
10. McEWEN, JA, ET AL: *Hazards associated with the use of disconnect monitors.* Anesthesiology 53:S391, September, 1980.
11. *Medical Device Alert #33. Failure to detect anaesthetic circuit disconnection.* Health Protection Branch Health and Welfare, Canada, January 15, 1981.
12. McEWEN, JA, SMALL, CF, JENKINS, LC: *A smart disconnect monitor for anaesthetic equipment.* In *Digest of the 8th Canadian Medical and Biological Engineers Conference,* 10-121, 1980.
13. RENDELL-BAKER, L AND MEYER, JA: *Accidental disconnection and pulmonary barotrauma.* Anesthesiology 58:286, 1983.
14. ANDERSON, CE AND RENDELL-BAKER, L: *Exposed O_2 flush hazard.* Anesthesiology 56:328, 1982.
15. *$Four Million Award Won in Suit Filed over 1980 Surgery. Huchingson v Little Rock Anesthesia Services and Airco Inc.* Report in *Arkansas Gazette,* September 18, 1981.
16. Dikran Agabanian v Juan Minelli. Pending in Los Angeles courts.
17. Canadian Standard Z168.4-1975: Keyed Filling Devices Applied to Anaesthetic Equipment.
18. KLEIN, SL AND CAMENIZIND, T: *Hazards of bottle adapters for vaporizers* Anesth Analg 57:596–597, 1978.
19. *Colour coding for classes of medicines used in anesthesiology.* South African Bureau of Standards Document dated 1/31/84, ISO/TC121 (Sec 148) N226.
20. *Dangerous mistakes in drug administration.* Medico-Pharmaceutical Forum Report, April, 1979. 1 Wimpole Street, London, W1M 8AE.
21. *Pantone Color Specifier—Designers' Edition of the Pantone Matching System.* Pantone, 55 Knickerbocker Road, Moonachie, NJ.
22. SMELLIE, GD, LEES, NW, SMITH EM: *Drug recognition by nurses and anaesthetists.* Anaesthesia 37:206–208, 1982.
23. IKEDA, S, SCHWEISS, JF: *Life-threatening similarity in drug packaging.* Anesthesiology 56:489–490, 1982.
24. FREUND, PR, WARD, RJ: *Drug packaging invites confusion.* Anethesiology 55:87–88, 1981.

APPENDIX A

Standards or Draft Standards of Interest to Anesthesiologists are available from the following organizations:

American National Standards Inc
1430 Broadway
New York, NY 10018
Contact: Susan Williams

Standards evolved by American National Standards Committee Z79 (sponsored by the American Society of Anesthesiologists)
Chairman: John Hedley-Whyte, M.D.
Beth Israel Hospital
330 Brookline Avenue, Boston, MA 02215
Secretary: Thomas C. Deas, M.D.
Temple University Health Sciences Center
3401 North Broad Street
Philadelphia, PA 19140

ANSI Number	Title of Standard
Z79.2-1976	Tracheal Tube Connectors and Adapters
Z79.3-1982	Oropharyngeal Airways and nasopharyngeal Airways
Z79.4-1974	Anesthetic Reservoir Bags*
Z79.6-1975	Breathing Tubes*
Z79.7-1976	Breathing Machines for Medical Use*
Z79.8-1979	Minimum Performance and Safety Requirements for Components and System of Continuous Flow Anesthesia Machines for Human Use.
Z79.9-1979	Humidifiers and Nebulizers
Z79.10-1979	Requirements for Oxygen Analyzers for Monitoring Direct Patient Breathing Mixtures

---

*New or revised draft standard under discussion. Information on these may be obtained from the secretary of the committee.

APPENDIX A—continued

Z79.11-1982	Anesthesia Gas Pollution Control
Z79.13-1981	Oxygen Concentrators
Z79.14-1982	Tracheal Tubes and Cuffs
Z79.XX	Terminology*
Z79.XX	Performance and Safety of Anesthesia Breathing Systems*
Z79.XX	Resuscitators*
Z79.XX	Cuffed Tracheal Tubes for Prolonged Use*
Z79.XX	Performance of Medical and Surgical Vacuum Systems*
Z79.XX	Cutaneous Oxygen Monitor*

Association for Advancement of Medical Instrumentation (AAMI)
Suite 602
1901 N. Ft. Myer Drive
Arlington, VA 22209
Contact: Judith Veale

Cardiovascular Devices

ANSI-AAMI-DF2-1981	American National Standard for Cardiac Defibrillator Devices
	Blood Transfusion Microfilters
ANSI-AAMI/AT6-1981	Autotransfusion Devices
	Blood Pressure Transducers—Resistive Bridge Type
	Cardiac Monitors, Heart Rate Meters and Alarm
	ECG Connectors
	Pregelled ECG Disposable Electrodes
	Nonautomated Sphygmomanometers
	Electronic or Automated Sphygmomanometers

Electrical Safety

AAMI-ESI Rev 1982	Proposed revised American National Standard, Safe Current Limits for Electromedical Apparatus

---

*New or revised draft standard under discussion. Information on these may be obtained from the secretary of the committee.

General Hospital Use
Infant Incubators
Infant Radiant Warmers
Infusion Devices
Intravenous Catheters or Cannulas

General Surgery
Electrosurgical Devices

Design Guidelines
Human Engineering Guidelines and Preferred Practices for Design of Medical Devices.

Neurosurgical/Neurology
Transcutaneous Electrical Nerve Stimulators
Peripheral Nerve Stimulators
Intracranial Pressure Monitoring Devices

Sterilization and Infection Control
Ethylene Oxide Sterilization—A Guide for Hospital Personnel
Good Hospital Practice: Ethylene Oxide Gas—Ventilation Recommendations and Safe Use
Good Hospital Practice: Steam Sterilization and Sterility Assurance
Hospital Steam Sterilizers
Test Methods for Determining Ethylene Oxide Residual Levels in Implantable Medical Devices

American Society for Testing and Materials (ASTM)
1916 Race Street
Philadelphia, PA 19103
Contact: Robert J. Morgan

Committee D10-34 Identification of Pharmaceutical Drug Product Containers
Recommended Practice—*Labels for Small Volume Parenteral (less than 100 ml) Drug Containers*

APPENDIX A—continued

Committee F 4 Medical and Surgical Materials and Devices

F469-78	Assessment of Compatibility of Non-Porous Polymeric Materials for Surgical Implants with Regard to Effect of Materials on Tissue
F640-79	Radiopacity of Plastics

Health Industry Manufacturers Association (HIMA)
1030 15th Street, N.W.
Washington, D.C. 20005
Contact: George Willingmyre
ANSI-MD70.1 Performance Standard for Medical Luer Taper Fittings

National Fire Protection Association (NFPA)
Batterymarch Park
Quincy, MA 02269
Contact: Burton Klein

Number	Title of Standard
NFPA-56A/1978	Standard for Use of Inhalation Anesthetics
ANSI/NFPA-56B	Standard on Respiratory Care (1976)
ANSI/NFPA-56F (1977)	Standard on Non-Flammable Medical Gas Systems
ANSI/NFPA-56G (1980)	Standard for Inhalation Anesthetics in Ambulatory Care Facilities
NFPA56HM	Manual of Home Use of Respiratory Therapy
NFPA-56K (1980)	Recommended Practice—Medical and Surgical Vacuum Systems
ANSI/NFPA-76Z (1977)	Standard for Essential Electrical Systems for Health Care Facilities
NFPA-76B/1980	Standard for the Safe Use of Electricity in Patient Care Areas of Hospitals
ANSI/NFPA-76C (1980)	Recommended Practice on Safe Use of High Frequency Electricity in Health Care Facilities

The Compressed Gas Association
1235 Jefferson Davis Highway
Arlington, VA 22202
Contact: Paul Mann
C-4   American National Standard Method of Marking Portable Compressed Gas Containers to Identify the Material Contained, ANSI Z48.1.
C-9   Standard Color-Marking of Compressed Gas Cylinders Intended for Medical Use in the United States
G-4   Oxygen
G-4.3   Commodity Specification for Oxygen
G-6   Carbon Dioxide
G-6.2   Commodity Specification for Carbon Dioxide
G-7   Compressed Air for Human Respiration
G-7.1   Commodity Specifications for Air
G-8.1   Standard for the Installation of Nitrous Oxide Systems at Consumer Sites
G-9.1   Commodity Specification for Helium
G-10.1   Commodity Specification for Nitrogen
M-1   Standard for 22 mm Anesthesia Breathing Circuit Connectors
P-2   Characteristics and Safe Handling of Medical Gases
P-2.1   Standard for Medical-Surgical Vacuum Systems in Hospitals
P-2.3T   Standard for Hyperbaric Facilities Intended for Use in Medical Application
P-4   Safe Handling of Cylinders by Emergency Rescue Squads
P-5   Suggestions for the Care of High-Pressure Air Cylinders for Underwater Breathing
P-6   Standard Density Data, Atmospheric Gases and Hydrogen

APPENDIX A—continued

V-1 American National-Canadian Standard Compressed Gas Cylinder Valve Outlet and Inlet Connections; ANSI-B57.1-1977 (includes the Pin Index System)

V-5 Diameter-Index Safety System

APPENDIX B

International Standards Organization (ISO)
1 Rue Varembe CHI-1111
Geneva 20, Switzerland

ISO/TC 121	*Anesthetic Equipment and Medical Breathing Machines*
Secretariat:	British Standards Institution
2 Park Street
London W1A 28S, England.
Contact:	Mr. A. Pittard
U.S. Contact:	American Society of Anesthesiologists

International Standards

ISO 5358-1980	Continuous Flow Inhalational Anaesthetic Apparatus for Use with Humans
ISO 5362-1980	Anaesthetic Reservoir Bags
ISO 5364-1980	Oropharyngeal Airways
ISO 5366/1-1980	Tracheostomy Tubes, Part I: Connectors
ISO 5367-1980	Breathing Tubes Used for Anaesthetic Apparatus and Ventilators

Draft International Standards

ISO/DIS 4135	Anaesthesiology and Medical Respirators—Vocabulary
ISO/DIS 5356/1	Breathing Attachments for Anesthetic Apparatus, Part I: Conical Fittings and Adapters
ISO/DIS 5356/2	Breathing Attachments for Anesthetic Apparatus, Part II: Screw Threaded Weight Bearing Fittings
ISO/DIS 5361/1	Tracheal Tubes, Part I: General Requirements
ISO/DIS 5361/2	Tracheal Tubes, Part II: Oral (plain and cuffed) and Nasal Tracheal Tubes—Magill Tubes

APPENDIX B—continued

ISO/DIS 5361/3	Tracheal Tubes, Part III: Murphy Tubes
ISO/DIS 5361/4	Tracheal Tubes, Part IV: Cole Tubes
ISO/DIS 5366/2	Tracheostomy Tubes, Part II: Basic Requirements
ISO/DIS 5369	Breathing Machines for Medical Use
ISO/DIS 7228	Tracheal Tube Connectors

Draft Proposals

ISO/DP 5359	Medical Gas Hose Assemblies
ISO/DP 5360	Keyed Filling Devices for Liquid Anesthetic Vaporizers
ISO/DP 5368	Equipment for Prolonged Tracheal Intubation
ISO/DP 7281	Anesthetic Gas Scavenging Systems
ISO/DP 7396	Medical Gas Pipeline Systems
ISO/DP 7481	Low-Pressure Flexible Connecting Assemblies for Use with Medical Gas Systems
ISO 32-1977 (E)	Gas Cylinders for Medical Use—Marking for Identification of Content
ISO-R 407	Yoke Type Valve Connections for Small Gas Cylinders and for Anesthetic Resuscitation Purposes

SECTION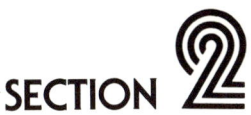

USING WHAT WE KNOW TO DESIGN FOR THE FUTURE

The following seven chapters address issues integral to anesthesia apparatus function. Implied is the fact that change from present standards is a necessity. The perturbations suggested are not futuristic speculations but, rather, recommendations predicated on available technology.

An anesthesia machine is basically a three-component model: 1) a source of anesthetic (compressed gas; vapor); 2) a monitor of anesthetic (flowmeter); and 3) a method of delivery of anesthetic (valves, tubing, and so forth). The authors have not really altered this basic system. Rather, they introduce concepts that either finely tune the basic components or provide the user with feedback capabilities which were not existent before. Monitoring anesthesia system gas concentrations is one example. For years anesthetics have been successfully delivered with only rudimentary knowledge on the part of the anesthetist as to the precise concentrations of each component pharmacologic administered. A few centers have attempted to overcome this lack of information with very expensive monitoring systems, primarily the mass spectrograph. Other centers have chosen to ignore the issue, deciding that the information is not absolutely necessary to the conduct of clinical anesthesia, or at least not from a cost-effective point of view. Immediate, comprehensible information about gases can enhance management of the difficult patient and can help prevent undetected system malfunction. The impact of an inexpensive, easily maintained, versatile, and rugged gas/vapor sensor on the discipline would be enormous. Closed-circuit anesthesia could be easily and safely employed, with all its salient virtues, with little need for cumbersome formulae. Another chapter discusses a technique currently available that may prove to be extremely useful: high-frequency ventilation. As indicated by the author, advantages such as a perfectly still brain for microneurosurgery and better oxygen delivery with reduced barotrauma are just around the corner.

Burnell R. Brown, Jr.

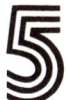

COMPONENTS OF THE SYSTEM: FUTURE DESIGN REQUIREMENTS

Jerry M. Calkins, Ph.D., M.D., and
Reynolds J. Saunders, M.D.

FUTURE CONCEPTS: A METHOD OF DEVELOPMENT

Mechanically, today's anesthesia machine is quite simple and extremely reliable. Unfortunately, this classic mechanical device is unwieldy for the user in today's operating room environment. In the usual situation, the machine is part of a large collection of unrelated pieces of apparatus surrounding the anesthetist and competing with the patient for attention.[1] Current machines tend to accrete multiple add-on devices of various functions, which may not even assist in the delivery of the anesthetic. Many of these unintegrated devices are electronic devices for physiologic monitoring (electrocardiograph, blood pressure transducers, thermocouples) and gas sensors (oxygen analyzers). For the most part, these systems are a hodgepodge of confusion and distractions for the user and risk to the patient through potential error.[1]

New technologies are available which can significantly add to sophistication of design but not necessarily to complexity and cost. Because automation, with simplicity, reliability, and versatility, is the direction of future technology, design will by necessity require both mechanical and electronic components, with appropriate interfacing. Both mechanical and electronic state-of-the-art technologies can be simple and reliable. Versatility will result from the number of system components and functions assigned to each. For example, it is quite possible to build a complete mechanical anesthesia system utilizing fluidic technology, with cost and function sacrificed in the areas of control, record keeping, and data acquisition and processing. Hence the necessity for mechanical-electronic hybrid systems employing electronic and mechanical components and utilizing the unique economics and benefits of each. Mechanically based systems with electronic control will also provide certain safety advantages.

Even with a paucity of human engineering and risk data concerning application and the integration of anesthesia delivery subsystems, some technologic improvement can begin immediately. Any design changes require the following steps: defining the function; specifying the requirements of the complete system, including various subsystems; critiquing currently utilized techniques; selecting appropriate state-of-the-art technology; and, finally, integrating the system into a functional unit. Critiques of current systems and the integration of the system are discussed in great detail in other chapters. This chapter will discuss the necessary functions and requirements of an anesthesia delivery system and provide insight into future design concepts and state-of-the-art technologies.

Defining the Function

Administration of general anesthesia to the patient involves delivering a variable combination of both respiratory gases (oxygen, nitrogen, air) and anesthetic gases (nitrous oxide, volatile anesthetics), and the administration of intravenous pharmacologic agents in sufficient amounts to produce a state in which the patient is unconscious and pain free and muscles are appropriately relaxed. Maintenance of the anesthetized state must continue throughout the operative procedure and must be easily reversed at the termination of surgery. The anesthetic procedure must be conducted quickly, safely, and with minimum stress for patient, surgeon, and anesthetist.

The process of anesthesia and thus function of any anesthesia delivery system is complex. However, it can be simplified into four phases: 1) setting parameters for delivery of the anesthetic agent(s), either general or regional; 2) monitoring perturbations by the anesthetic of the patient's physiologic variables; 3) intervening in the patient's altered physiologic processes with appropriate therapeutic adjuncts, such as fluids and drugs; and 4) surveillance of the process, with sufficient record keeping to document events and patient status.[2]

Although they are important components of any anesthesia delivery system, patient-monitoring techniques, decision-making processes, intervention methodologies, and record keeping will not be considered here. For the purposes of this discussion, only the techniques for the delivery of general anesthetic agents will be considered.

Requirements

Any delivery system must meet the patient's varying requirements for respiratory and anesthetic gases accurately and safely. The system must be able to deliver general anesthesia by any of a number of techniques accepted by the anesthesia community. This must be accomplished regardless of the breathing system chosen by the anesthetist. That is, the machine must have the capability to meet the demands of either a nonrebreathing or a partial rebreathing system. Today this includes high-flow open loop (semiclosed without absorber), low flow (semiclosed with carbon dioxide absorber), and closed circuit.

The system must have some capability of monitoring the effect of anesthesia upon the patient and the function of the delivery system itself. Monitoring should include estimation of drug absorbed by the patient. Another consideration is frequent and complete documentation of both this monitoring process and any actions taken.

The clear direction for the future is automation of some components, with improved economics, surveillance, and predictability. The concept of such a system, with the necessary subsystem components, is diagrammed in Figure 1. These include 1) gas supply and proportioning system; 2) volatile anesthetic delivery; 3) the breathing circuit, including anesthetic recovery, humidification, and carbon dioxide absorber; 4) sensors; 5) ventilator; and 6) the computer, with appropriate inputs and outputs for integration of the machine-anesthesiologist-patient relationships.

Gas Proportionating Systems

Commercially available anesthetic gas delivery systems are less than adequate, in part because of multiple deficiencies found in the flowmeters. The most widely and commonly used flowmeter type is the rotameter. Although simplistic in operation, this type of variable orifice

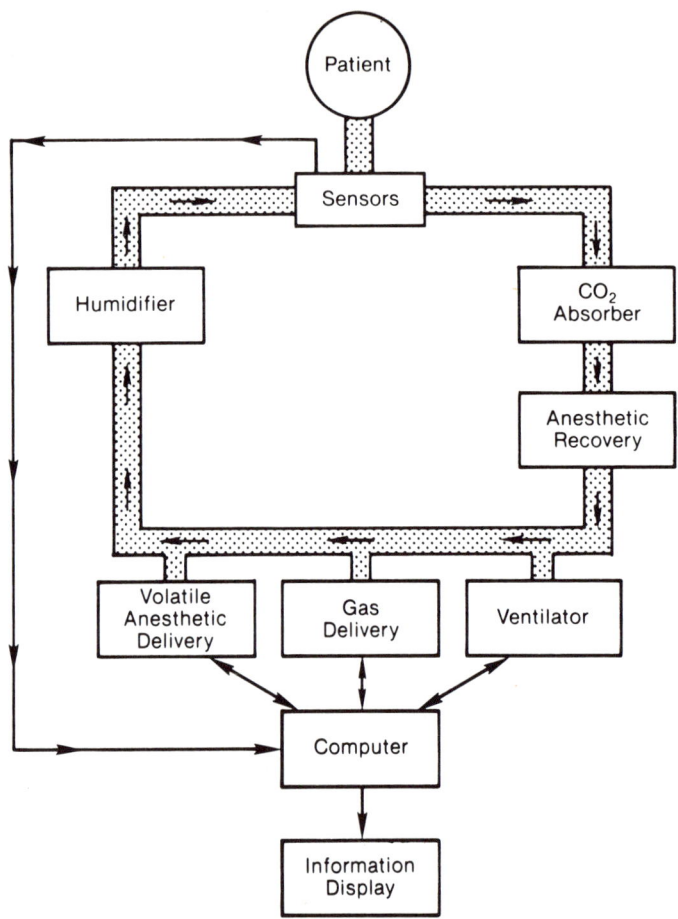

Figure 1. The anesthesia circuit is the organizing framework into which other elements of the system are integrated.

flow metering/measuring device is fraught with problems. These problems include inaccuracies produced by dirt and clogging of the rotameter tubes; the effects of back pressure from the breathing system; improper alignment of the flowmeters; indicators hiding at the top of the tube; blockage of the flowmeter at the tube outlet; and the effects of static electricity upon the bobbin. A recent study made on the accuracies of flowmeters used in vaporizers indicates that, when compared with highly reliable and precise linear resistor flowmeters, errors in accuracy of flowmeters in routine clinical use ranged from 10 percent to 20 percent, with errors as high as 50 percent.[3] In addition to the mechanical problems of the variable orifice rotameter, this particular type of flow device is not easily converted to automatic control, whether with needle valves or diaphragm-operated valving systems.

It appears that newer technologies in flowmeter and gas-proportionating design need to be considered. Any gas-delivery system needs to enable the operator to select accurate flows under varying external conditions. If the anesthetist chooses to use high-flow systems (1 to 10 liters per minute for gases), then the system should enable this to be done. However, because the trend is toward low-flow (0 to 1 liter per minute) and closed systems, then consideration should be given to dual-flow ranges. In addition, a high-flow, or bypass, system providing from 35 to 75 liters per minute oxygen will also be necessary. With these specifications in mind, what are the potentials? Fluidic technology with linear orifice flowmeters, vortex flowmeters, and a variety of other accurate, reliable measurement techniques are readily available. In addition to these, electromechanical gas-control devices with appropriate timing and valving arrangements have also been evaluated.

Volatile Anesthetic Delivery Systems

More precise and flexible control of the processes occurring within an anesthesia system is required in order to employ techniques that consider the uptake and distribution of anesthetic agents. One important process is volatile anesthetic delivery. Currently available techniques have significant problems which produce erratic and unpredictable delivery of vapor. Temperature variations, corrosion and plugging of the vaporizers, and back pressures in the circuits may all affect vapor delivery. Inability to prevent wrong anesthetics from being placed in the vaporizers is another hazard. In addition, large diluent gas flows are required for accurate delivery of a concentration of vapor.

Because of the physical properties of the volatile liquids, each requires a minimum thermal energy to obtain vapor pressures sufficient for the ranges of concentrations necessary for appropriate levels of anesthesia. Hence, newer techniques, such as activated syringe pump injectors and fluidic atomizers, are easily and safely controlled, and they deliver concentrations with higher accuracies than commercial units. With better control and more accurate delivery systems, anesthetics can be directly injected into the circuit, as opposed to gas bypass vaporizers. This technique then will enable the operator to control more precisely amounts (mass of) vapor delivered to the patient.

Breathing Circuit

The complete breathing circuit of future systems must have the capabilities for humidification, carbon dioxide absorption, anesthetic waste scavenging, and various assorted sensors to provide information regarding the operation and control of the system. The necessity for humidification and carbon dioxide removal has been well documented and investigated.

Numerous investigations have been made involving the effects of anesthetic gas exposure upon congenital birth defects and the carcinogenicity of these agents. Although the data are inconclusive at this time, sufficient information exists within some animal studies to make it highly suggestive that these agents have potential for creating undesired effects. However, in addition to the effects found within the operating room, consideration must be given to the effects of volatile agents, such as nitrous oxide, being dumped into the atmosphere; the potential for destruction of the ozone layer and other effects exist. The cost savings might be such that recovery of nitrous oxide would justify small recovery units for each hospital, so that this agent could be recycled and used more efficiently.

Sensors

Various types of sensors located within the machine and circuit, as well as in the patient, will be required in anesthesia delivery systems of the future. These sensors will provide the three basic functions of vigilance monitoring, control of anesthetic depth, and physiologic assessment. In order to accomplish these functions, the sensor will detect changes or magnitudes in the variable being monitored and provide the necessary inputs to either the anesthetist and/or microprocessor controller. In either case, the data provided by the sensor will be analyzed, processed, and integrated into decision making by the anesthetist.

A major type of sensor for future systems is the gas sensor, which can identify and analyze the concentrations of various respiratory and anesthetic gases found within the gas machine and patient circuit. Gas sensors can be used to determine average concentrations in both inspiratory and expiratory limbs of the circuit, and they can provide single-breath, end-tidal exhaled gas concentrations for estimation of a level or gas concentration as an indicator of anesthetic depth. With immediate results of this analysis available, vigilance monitoring can assist in the prevention of a critical incident by providing necessary information to the anesthetist about machine performance and patient status. The anesthetist can be alerted to both gradual and catastrophic changes in gas conditions. By precise measurement of the concentrations of gaseous anesthetic agents, the depth of anesthesia can be more easily controlled. In addition, the functional status of the cardiovascular and respiratory systems, such as physiologic dead space and cardiac output, may be obtained by incorporation of other variables measured by other sensors and simple calculations done by the system's computer.

In addition to gas concentration sensors, machine and circuit sensors indicating flow and pressure within the system will also assist in vigilance and surveillance. Evidence of appropriate flows (average and rate per minute) and system pressures will serve to verify proper function and performance. These will certainly increase patient safety by detecting disconnections and overpressurization.

Microprocessor Control

Because the wave of the future is toward automation, the heart of the new anesthesia delivery system will be a microcomputer and the various components that are necessary to interface it with the rest of the system. Various sensors will provide data input as well as receive input from the anesthetist. This information will be processed and assembled in such a manner that data will be displayed to the anesthetist as unambiguous physiologic variables; alarms will sound in hazardous situations; and second-to-second adjustments will be made in operation via actuators to make the appropriate concentration changes or ventilatory changes to maintain the anesthetist's treatment plan. In addition, microprocessors will lend themselves very easily and simply to interfacing a number of electronic components, which will provide the capability for accurate, partially automatic record keeping.

A microprocessor will be utilized for controlled automatic regulation of anesthetic gases and vapor delivery. The data put into the microprocessor will be from gas concentration and flow rate sensors, which continuously monitor the patient's inhaled and exhaled gases; and from keyboard-entered data, such as anesthetic drug codes, patient body mass, and so forth. Most importantly, the anesthetist will specify how the system should function. The microprocessor will have the ability to compare the actual system delivery variables with the preprogrammed anesthesia plan data. The output signal from the microprocessor will be sent to controllers regulating the gas-proportionating and volatile liquid anesthetic delivery systems. At any time during the course of the anesthetic administration, the anesthetist may modify the theoretic uptake track or may change to a manual mode of operation, thereby overriding all automatic control. Additional features also being investigated and developed as modular components are visual displays, volatile liquid recovery systems, ventilators, voice recognition devices, synthetic voice annunciators, anesthesia record printers, urine output monitors, and muscle relaxant infusion control systems.

Ventilators

Many anesthetized patients have their homeostatic control of arterial carbon dioxide impaired by anesthetics or muscle relaxants. Assessment and control of ventilation is an integral part of the anesthetic delivery process. Any really serviceable design must allow for rebreathing and closed-system techniques, must be amenable to automatic control through data from gas sensors, and must provide physiologic parameter control similar to that of ventilators used in critical care units.

For the apneic patient, the ventilator is the mechanical means, easily accessible to the anesthesiologist, that provides the artificial method of ventilating the patient. It must be effectively integrated into the system in such a manner that the change from spontaneous to mechanical ventilation can occur simply. Appropriate sensors need to be incorporated to provide operational, safety, and physiologic information.

Two concepts for its integration into the system exist. The first is commonly used in this country and considers the ventilator an accessory to the machine. This simplifies the design of the delivery system and easily enables the incorporation of low-flow closed-circuit delivery with rebreathing of gases (minus carbon dioxide). The second concept appears to be more popular in Europe. In this concept, the anesthesia system is built around the ventilator. This approach may complicate the design of function with emphasis toward high-flow rather than low-flow delivery.

Whether currently used, conventional ventilation will continue or newer modes, such as high-frequency ventilation, will be included only time will tell. However, any system design should be flexible enough to allow for change and should be modular to allow options to be installed as desired.

SUMMARY

A few ideas about future design concepts have been outlined and highlighted. Whether anesthetists will accept it or not, automation is the direction of the future, and data processing is increasingly important. Anesthesiology and industry need to initiate total cooperative efforts for appropriate implementation of modern technology.

REFERENCES

1. NEWBOWER, RS, COOPER, JB, TRAUTMAN, ED: *A microprocessor-based anesthesia delivery system.* In EDEN, HS AND EDEN, M (EDS): *Microcomputers in Patient Care.* Noyes Medical Publications, 158–173, 1981.
2. MYLREA, KC, ET AL: *Automated anesthesia delivery and patient management in the operating room.* In KARNI, S (ED): *24th Midwest Symposium on Circuits and Systems.* University of New Mexico Press, 1981, pp 667–673.
3. SAUNDERS, RJ, CALKINS, JM, GOODIN, TG: *Accuracy of rotameters and linear flowmeters.* Anesthesiology (Supp) 55:A116, 1981.

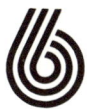

GAS AND VAPOR DELIVERY

Jerry M. Calkins, Ph.D., M.D.,
Reynolds J. Saunders, M.D., and
Charles K. Waterson, B.S.E.

One of the most important functions of any anesthesia system is the delivery of respiratory (oxygen, nitrogen/air) and anesthetic (nitrous oxide, volatile agents) gases. These gases must be delivered to the patient safely and reliably at precisely known and controlled concentrations and flow rates. This delivery requirement must be accomplished regardless of the type of technique employed by the anesthetist: high-flow (open or semiclosed), at total flow rates varying from 3 to 10 liters per minute; low-flow (semiclosed), at rates ranging from 500 ml per minute to 2 liters per minute; and the completely closed circuit, in which flow based upon patient requirements may be as low as 5 to 10 ml per minute for the pediatric patient, increasing to 200 to 1000 ml per minute for the adult. In each of these flow ranges, a closely controlled concentration of volatile anesthetic must be available. In addition to metered flows, arrangements must be made to meet high-flow oxygen "flush" requirements ranging from 35–75 liters per minute.[1]

IDEAL GAS AND VAPOR DELIVERY SYSTEM

Safe delivery of respiratory and anesthetic gases requires precise control, which must be accomplished through accurate measurement and regulation of the rate of mass flow of the various constituent gases into the patient circuit. Because of the number of independent variables involved, the end result of this delivery process can be expressed two ways. The first method, termed "flow proportionate gas delivery," controls concentration and total flow independently. The other method, referred to as "gas mixing," controls the flow rate of each constituent independently to produce the desired concentration and consequently total flow.

Gas mixing is the technique utilized in all current anesthesia machines. The rate of mass delivery of each constituent is independently controlled and measured by needle valves and rotameters. The final concentration and total flow rate determined by mixing these component flows are dependent functions and subject to the accuracy of the control and measurement equipment.

In a proportionating system, the delivered concentration of each gas constituent is a function of a predetermined, precisely controlled ratio of proportionality, independent of the total flow of gas involved. For example, if a final mixture of 70 percent nitrous oxide and 30 percent oxygen is required, the metered rate of mass delivery of nitrous oxide and oxygen will always be in a ratio of 7:3, regardless of the total flow rate. Hence, concentration is only a function of setting the proportional relationship between constituents rather than setting individual gas flows.

The significance of the differences between these two gas delivery techniques is more apparent once an understanding of a few simple physical principles is obtained. First is the principle of conservation of mass, which states that the rate of mass flowing into a system (patient) normally must equal the rate of mass flowing from the system (patient). If these rates are not equal, the difference between the two must be accounted for by either accumulation (storage-uptake) or reaction (metabolism). In other words, what goes in must come out or accumulate or react. Therefore, every anesthesia delivery system and technique must provide a means of getting a quantity (mass) of gas (respiratory and anesthetic) into and out of a patient, with a minimal amount of unnecessary accumulation and at a sufficient rate to meet various anesthetic and physiologic requirements.

From the conservation of mass, the total mass flow rate (ω_t) into the circuit must equal the sum of the individual mass flow rates of each constituent (ω_i). For a binary mixture, such as nitrous oxide and oxygen, this can be expressed mathematically as

$$(1) \quad \omega_t = \omega_1 + \omega_2$$

This mass balance equation contains three variables. Hence, if two of the three variables are known, the third is defined. For example, if ω_1 and ω_2 are selected as in gas mixing, the total mass flow rate is determined. Or, as in gas proportionating, if total flow rate and the proportionality ratio (ω_1/ω_2) are defined, then the flow rate of each constituent is determined.

Ideally, the various rates of mass flow need to be measured and controlled. However, from a practical point of view this may not be that simple. Fortunately, for a gas at the usual conditions of pressure and temperature of routine anesthesia delivery, the amount of mass can be related to system volume and pressure by use of the ideal gas law, and the rate of mass flow (mass/time) is a function of volumetric flow rate (volume/time) at system pressure and temperature.

Therefore, if the system pressure, temperature, and volumetric flow rates are measured, the mass flow rate can be determined. Unfortunately, because of the interrelationship between volume, pressure, and temperature, significant error in measurement and interpretation can be made if only volumes are used.[1,2]

Ideal Flowmeter

Regardless of the delivery technique, flow measurement requires a gas flowmeter that ideally measures the rate of mass flow rather than a volumetric flow because anesthetic induction is determined by mass uptake, not volume. This mass flow rate measurement should be accomplished independently of the characteristics of the gas constituents (viscosity, density) flowing through it. The ideal flowmeter measures flows with minimal compression of gas volume and is independent of system temperature and pressure. Ideally, these measurements should be accomplished with a single flowmeter, having sufficient range and adequate resolution for both low-flow and high-flow techniques. An adequately fast time response and an electronic output should be provided to allow for interfacing with a computerized control system. Depending upon the design, this flowmeter can be used as either a flow indicator (showing approximate flow rates of the constituents) or in controlling flow (when actual flow metering is required, such as in closed-circuit anesthesia).

Ideal Vapor Delivery

Inasmuch as several general anesthetic agents are volatile liquids, these compounds must be converted into vapors before delivery to the anesthetic circuit. In order to accomplish this, the thermal energy level of the liquid must be sufficiently increased to produce vaporization. Because the process requires heat transfer and is a strong function of liquid temperature, an ideal vaporizer will prevent a decrease in liquid temperature and will provide efficient heat transport. Hence, consideration of materials with high specific heats and thermal conductivities is essential for a vapor delivery system.[1]

GAS DELIVERY

Current Techniques of Gas Delivery

At present, compressed gas enters the anesthesia machine via hospital supply lines or from storage cylinders attached to the machine. Gas supplied by the hospital is usually maintained at a pressure ranging between 40 and 50 psi. Gas from cylinders is regulated via machine pressure regulators to approximately this same pressure.

From the supply source, the gas is directed through a flow delivery unit which usually consists of a rotameter and a needle valve; one delivery unit is used with each gas regulated. The units are connected in parallel and exhaust into a common manifold prior to leaving the machine.

Although simple in design and function, this flow delivery unit is far from the ideal system, owing to a number of performance-related problems.[1] Needle valves are prone to both leakage and looseness around the stem packing. The closing interface between the needle tip of the valve stem and its seat is prone to leak as a result of wear. The control knobs may come loose, or they may be positioned in such a manner that accidental bumping, with inappropriate flow alteration, may occur.

Rotameters also are fraught with mechanical and operational problems. The flow indicators (bobbins, floats) are prone to stick unless the glass tubes are immaculately clean and free of static electricity. Over time the flowmeters tend to become inaccurate. A recent study evaluated accuracy of the low-range flowmeters (0 to 500 ml per minute) on anesthesia machines in clinical use (routinely serviced for preventive maintenance); the rotameter reading varied as much as 50 percent from true flow.[2] In addition, the design of current gas delivery systems allows inaccuracies of flow produced by density changes in the gas; this error occurs when back pressure from either obstruction or ventilator cycling is transmitted to the flowmeters from the circuit.

This effect is commonly referred to as the "bounding or bouncing bobbin." Other problems, including bobbins hidden at the top of the tube and improper vertical alignment, may also lead to inaccuracies.

For the most part, with the exception of certain ANSI Z79 recommendations, current anesthesia machines do not have appropriate safety features. Early machines had "oxygen failure safety valves," which were master pressure regulators. These controlled slave pressure/flow regulators were located in the nitrous oxide line. Pure nitrous oxide could be delivered with only oxygen supply pressure present; no oxygen flow was required. More recent machines (as a result of Z79 standards), through ingenious mechanical linkages, pressure-repeating diaphragm units, and other various mechanical devices, do not allow delivery of gas mixtures with oxygen concentration below a lower limit of at least 20 percent (usually higher) and a continuous flow of oxygen of at least 200 ml per minute when the machine is in a standby mode. This type of gas delivery may be quite sufficient for the anesthetist who prefers high-flow techniques and is not concerned with economy of gas utilization. Unfortunately, this technique is quite unsatisfactory for the individual desiring closed-circuit or low-flow techniques, both because of the high minimum flow rates and because gas concentration delivered to the circuit corresponds poorly to inspired concentration at low flows.

In addition, current delivery techniques are not readily adaptable to electronic surveillance or control because of rotary controls, imprecision of needle valves, and lack of electronic feedback about flow rates. Automatic control of flow, with feedback from the needle valves for flow regulation, is simply not practical with current designs.

Future Techniques of Gas Delivery

The initial step in designing a gas delivery system is to consider the system requirements and what technology is available that most closely will enable development of the "ideal" gas delivery system. Although some design criteria may seem idealistic, technology exists today that can solve many of the problems of current systems.

FLOWMETERS

The rotameter is classified as a variable orifice flowmeter. It consists of a tapered transparent (glass) tube whose internal diameter increases from bottom to top. The tube contains a flow indicator, or bobbin, whose position is directly related to the flow rate. Because the pressure drop across a given rotameter is constant, the reading is dependent upon the variable flow area of the tapered tube. Because of the operational and design characteristics of the rotameter, the numerous problems created by back pressure, temperature, and other features previously discussed are difficult to correct. Fortunately, many of the current flowmeter problems can be overcome by simple fluidic components that can be integrated efficiently into fluidic-electronic hybrid systems.

One type of fluidic flowmeter is the linear resistance laminar flowmeter (LRLF). Gas flow is determined with the LRLF by measuring the differential pressure produced as a gas flows over a given distance through a channel that produces laminar flow. The differential pressure across a standard distance in the laminar flow path is linearly proportional to the flow rate. This device has an accuracy of better than 1 percent of full scale when used within a defined range of flow rates. Pressure can be measured both visually, using differential pressure gauges, or electronically, using differential pressure transducers. The ability to measure the flow electronically provides the capability of feedback control of gas flow rates and concentrations. As with the rotameters, this technique requires correction for back pressure, temperature, and changes in gas characteristics when the same device is used with other gas constituents.

Besides the LRLF, other common industrial techniques such as pitot tubes, venturi meters, and fixed orifice devices are also available for consideration. The pitot tube measures the velocity at a point, which can be related to a volume or mass flow rate if the conduit areas and characteristics of the gas are known. The venturi and orifice devices measure an average velocity as a function of pressure drop and can be used in a manner similar to the pitot tube. One of the serious disadvantages of average velocity devices is that a large percentage of the pressure drop is not recoverable, hence higher operating pressures are required. Also, these devices are once again volume flowmeters requiring corrections for temperature, pressure, and gas characteristics. Some specialized mass flowmeters, such as thermal techniques, are available but have not been investigated for use in anesthesia delivery systems.

FLOW CONTROLLERS

Flow can be *controlled* by numerous electronic or fluidic valves (which do not suffer from the problems of needle valves); these include fluidic valves, time-controlled electromechanical valves, and binary valve arrays.[3]

One type of fluidic device that has been designed for application as a flow controller is the flueric vortex valve. A vortex valve utilizes a small low-pressure control gas flow (oxygen) introduced tangentially into a flowing power stream (oxygen, nitrous oxide) coming from a high-pressure source to throttle the flow. The centrifugal forces that are introduced by the tangential flow cause an increase in impedance, leading to a decrease in flow rate.

An example of the time-controlled type is a fixed orifice with a fixed flow, controlled by a solenoid. The overall flow rate is controlled by the fraction of time gas is allowed to flow through the orifice. Pulsatile flow can be easily smoothed (if necessary) by mechanical techniques, varying from a simple storage tank to more complex diaphragm pressure systems.

Another electromechanical flow control scheme is the array of binary valves.[3] In this technique, several fixed orifice valves (usually eight) are arranged in parallel. The fixed orifice of each valve in the parallel array is larger than the one next to it and provides a flow rate that is a power of two greater. If the flow through the first valve is 10 ml per minute when it is on, the flow through the eighth valve would be 1280 ml per minute when it is on. By opening and closing valves in combination, 255 discrete total flows can be obtained with the resolution of the smallest valve. These binary valves are easily adapted to direct computer control.

In addition to these three techniques, many other flow control techniques have been used in industrial applications. A few may be more suitable for incorporation into the anesthesia delivery system than others. However, they are already available as alternatives to the present needle-valve and rotameter system.

GAS MIXING AND PROPORTIONATING

The gas mixing function can be accomplished easily with any combination of flowmeters and control valves previously mentioned. Gas proportionating can be easily accomplished using commercially available pressure-balanced gas blenders. In addition to these, new fluidic techniques utilizing jet entrainment, venturi aspiration, and vortex proportionating valves should be considered. With each of these, the problems of temperature and pressure sensitivity and flow control valve regulation are not significant, because control of delivery results from system pressure regulation.

VAPOR DELIVERY

Another integral portion of the gas delivery system is introduction of the volatile anesthetic drug. Volatile anesthetic agents must be converted from a liquid to a gaseous phase at an appropriate rate to produce either a defined inspired or end-tidal concentration or a given mass delivery rate.

Conversion of a liquid to a gas requires energy. The greater the amount of energy, the greater the rate of vaporization. For volatile agents, this energy is supplied in the form of heat. The amount of heat required depends upon the heat of vaporization and the specific heat of the anesthetic. The larger these factors, the greater the amount of heat required. Fortunately, heat requirements are low enough that sufficient heat can be supplied from the ambient surroundings in the operating suite. The maximum concentration that can be delivered from standard vaporizers is mainly a function of vaporizer temperature and is reflected in the vapor pressure of the anesthetic agent at the given temperature.

The basic design of a vaporizer should be quite simple. The liquid must be housed in a closed container, and enough energy must be applied to vaporize it. As the liquid is vaporized, the resultant gas must be exhausted and must be injected into the patient's breathing circuit. This can be accomplished by an in-line device (in the patient circuit) or out-of-line (in parallel with the breathing circuit).[1]

Current Techniques of Vapor Delivery

Common techniques include variable-bypass, wick-type vaporizers, or bubble-through vaporizers that are dependent upon rotameters for their accuracy. With these current designs, either in-line or out-of-line, several basic design problems exist.[1] Many systems still enable the delivery of more than one agent at a time. Recent Z79 recommendations call for interlocking vaporizers to prevent this. All current vaporizers possess efficiency problems resulting from corrosion, scaling, and fouling resulting from long-term use.[1] Many designs are not flow, temperature, or pressure compensated, and they change delivery characteristics when any of these variables changes. Several designs allow mixing of agents in the same vaporizer.

Future Techniques of Vapor Delivery

Any design for vaporization in future delivery systems must overcome these problems of variability in delivery as well as in safety. Again, both fluidic and electromechanical technologies offer distinctive solutions to these problems. Energy can be supplied easily by accessory heaters or various types of heat exchanges. Mass administration rates can be controlled by volumetric liquid injection through atomizers into the circuit or into vaporizers for mixing with the gas stream. Agents can be keyed to be unambiguously identified for supply to appropriate vaporizer units. Superior technology exists for vaporization that is neither complex nor expensive.

SUMMARY

Technology for gas and vapor delivery has not changed substantively in decades. Technology possessing greater precision and reliability has been in use by nonmedical industries to regulate gas flows and to vaporize liquids. Adaptation of existing technology to the needs of anesthesia delivery systems requires stimulus from the anesthesia community and commitment from the anesthesia device industry. No insurmountable problems are evident, but the perennial problem of inertia has prevented progress consistent with that seen in other fields of biomedical technology.

REFERENCES

1. Dorsch, JA and Dorsch, SE: *Understanding Anesthesia Equipment: Construction Care and Complications.* Williams & Wilkins, Baltimore, 1975, pp 42–56, 84–88.
2. Saunders, RJ, Calkins, JM, Goodin, TM: *Accuracy in rotameters and linear flowmeters.* Anesthesiology (Suppl) 55:A116, 1981.
3. Cooper, JB, et al: *A new anesthesia delivery system.* Anesthesiology 49:310–318, 1978.

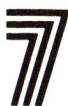

RECOVERY OF WASTE ANESTHETIC GASES
Charles K. Waterson, B.S.E.

In the past few years, attention has been paid to the problem of chronic exposure to waste anesthetic gases in the operating room. Although the seriousness of the health hazard caused by this exposure is a question at issue, the consensus is that waste gases should be scavenged and removed from the operating suite. However, an assumption made in dealing with these waste gases was that they had no effect on the atmosphere or environment outside the hospital. Unfortunately, this is not true. Not only is there reason to be concerned with the presence of detritus vapors in the immediate vicinity of the anesthetist and operating room staff, but evidence exists of potential harm to the atmosphere by waste anesthetics.

Little consideration has been given to the manufacturing costs of inhalation anesthetics and respiratory gases. It is assumed that this cost is negligible. Perhaps that is so on an individual patient basis, especially when compared to costs of some other drugs, equipment, or professional charges, but when the perspective is widened to that of the institution, practice group, or patient population, the cost is not insignificant and should be reduced.

How can the expenditures for inhalation anesthetics and respiratory gases be reduced and the environmental impact be lessened? Obviously, one way is to use less. Low-flow/closed-circuit anesthesia has already proven efficacious, safe, and may have additional benefits in clinical management of the patient. Techniques can be modified to use more fixed intravenous agents. However, intravenous anesthetics are not without drawbacks. Nor can closed-circuit anesthesia be used for every single case. An alternative that has not been fully explored, and is proposed in this chapter, is the approach of scavenging the exhaled gases, separating the components, and recycling them for anesthetic and respiratory use. This approach could not only remove excess anesthetic gases from the operating room environment but could provide additional economic and ecologic benefits.

To provide a framework within which this option can be explored and its advantages and disadvantages understood, it is beneficial to define three interrelated systems and delineate some of the effects of the inhalation anesthetic agents within each frame of reference. The three systems to be considered are the patient, the operating room, and the atmosphere surrounding planet earth. The impact of the waste anesthetics in the operating room and atmosphere are summarized, and guidelines are discussed for effective scavenging. Theoretical processes are proposed for separation and reclamation of anesthetics. The potential costs and benefits of adopting such a plan are also discussed.

EFFECTS OF ANESTHETIC GASES IN THREE CONCENTRIC SYSTEMS

The anesthesiologist practices within several concentric environments (Fig. 1). The immediate environment is the operating room, but there are also larger systems in which the operating room is but a small component. Humans have long attempted to control their immediate surroundings by heat, light, cooling, visual stimulus, sound, and physical arrangement; but they have often been neglectful of their impact upon the larger ecosystem which exists just outside our walls. One example of this is the impact of waste anesthetic gases in the operating room and in the ecosystem. The accumulation of vapors in either system can be a problem, but the majority of efforts have been aimed at removing gases from the operating room, that is, simply shifting the concentration to the atmosphere outside the hospital, where it is diluted. Although this certainly reduces accumulation in one system, it is not without significance in the other system, namely, the atmosphere.

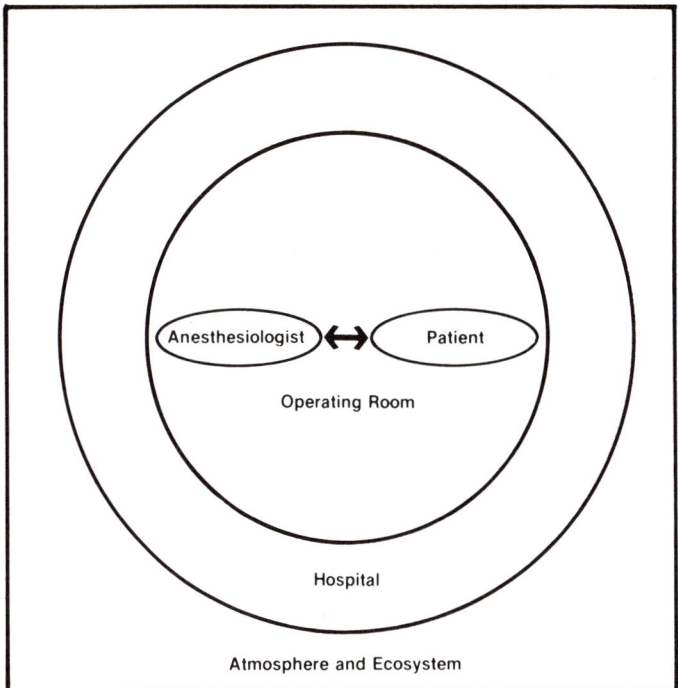

Figure 1. The anesthesiologist interacts with several systems.

System One: The Patient

Before a change can be made in how used anesthetic vapors are handled, the reason and method for their introduction into the operating room (OR) environment must be considered. Obviously the intended purpose of inhalation agents is for anesthesia. In order for that to occur, a sufficient amount of agent must enter the patient's blood. However, most of the anesthetic inhaled in any given breath is exhaled without being taken up or "consumed" by the patient. Because only the agent taken up will have any effect, the exhaled agent is wasted.

The premise in closed-circuit anesthesia is that this exhaled agent will be reintroduced repeatedly until the patient is in equilibrium with the breathing circuit input. In that case, no waste would exit the breathing circuit and there would be no concern about anesthetic vapors in the operating room air. However, most anesthesiologists do not use closed-circuit techniques, and there are some cases in which they cannot be used. Also, when the time comes for the patient to emerge from anesthesia, the anesthetic must be allowed to exit the system via the breathing circuit.

So, no matter what inhalation technique is used, some anesthetic gas must become waste and move from the system of the patient into the operating room environment. A few anesthetic techniques waste more agent than others, but all contribute something. Inasmuch as waste anesthetics pass the boundary between the patient and the outside world, the effects of the waste gases in these outside systems must be considered.

System Two: Waste Anesthetics in the Operating Room

Much discussion and study have been devoted in recent years to the hazards of exposure to waste anesthetics in the operating room, recovery room, and dental offices.[1-4] It would be presumptuous of me to pretend to have any extra insight into the continuing controversy over the extent of this hazard.[5-7] However, a conservative approach is favored, and so a listing of suggested effects, without comment as to validity or scientific merit of studies producing these results, will be presented. A critical review of the literature is outside the scope of this chapter.

The effects of chronic exposure to waste anesthetics can be categorized as psychomotor effects, increased rates of spontaneous abortion, increased rates of birth defects, carcinogenicity, and hepatic or renal disease.[1] Other effects have been associated with exposure to low levels of halothane, such as increased drug metabolism,[8] but these findings are inconclusive. It must be noted that most of the effects listed have been found through retrospective epidemiologic studies. The validity of the findings of such a study is dependent on establishing a suitable control group for comparison. Because of stress and other work-related factors for medical personnel working in operating rooms, it is difficult to define a control comparison population and to establish cause-and-effect relationships between the listed effects and prolonged exposure to low levels of waste anesthetics. However, the consensus is that there is sufficient evidence for concern. In any case, it is relatively simple to reduce risk by reducing exposure.

By virtue of the way inhalation anesthetics are administered, a certain level of these drugs will be introduced into the operating room environment. These waste anesthetic gases come from two sources, influenced by the technique and equipment being used. The first source is that of leaks in the equipment and breathing circuit. This source can be reduced by routine preventive maintenance and careful checking of the machine and circuit before use. Further reductions can be accomplished by modification of technique to insure that anesthetics are turned off whenever the breathing circuit is disconnected, mask fit is adequate, and that tracheal tube cuffs do not leak.

The largest portion of anesthetic waste, however, is produced by the technique of semiclosed, high-flow anesthesia. Although the circuits commonly in use are supposedly rebreathing semiclosed systems, the typical gas flow through such a system is on the order of 5 liters per minute. This is in contrast to the actual metabolic needs of the patient and uptake rate for any anesthetic. Indeed, a typical adult may need only 200 to 300 ml oxygen per minute and take up an almost insignificant amount of anesthetic. It can readily be seen that the majority of respiratory and anesthetic gases are breathed in once by the patient, reside in the lung for a brief period of time, then are exhaled and ultimately exhausted from the breathing circuit. This constant outflow of oxygen, carbon dioxide, and anesthetic gases through ventilator and breathing circuit pop-off valves must be dealt with in some way. If they are uncollected, they will concentrate in the room air. Although operating rooms are typically well ventilated with nonrecirculating air conditioning systems, the flow rate of air through the room is inadequate to keep accumulated concentration of the waste anesthetics to a low level. Also, not all areas are ventilated with totally nonrecirculated air because of energy cost constraints.

This has led to several active scavenging systems which remove the waste anesthetics directly from the ventilator or breathing circuit pop-off valve and exhaust them from the room. In most cases these systems have proven to be effective in lowering operating room concentrations of the waste anesthetics. However, evidence does not exist to allow a determination of exactly what levels are safe for those anesthetics in the operating room. Instead, the recommended exposure levels (25 ppm for nitrous oxide, 2 ppm for any halogenated anesthetic agent) are based on the lowest levels that can be achieved by a scavenging system without undue impairment on technique or requiring expensive equipment.[4]

Optimum conditions for scavenging the operating room environment have previously been defined.[4,9-13] The key aspects of waste removal that contribute to maximum efficiency include an active scavenging system, generally of the high-flow/low-vacuum design, a leakproof gas supply and anesthesia machine, a closed and regularly maintained anesthesia breathing circuit, and an adequate level of ventilation within the room. Ventilation should be well distributed as well as have an adequate rate of nonrecirculating air exchange.

As previously mentioned, the technique of the anesthesiologist in administering the anesthetic affects the efficiency of these scavenging systems. In order for the gases to be removed from the operating room environment, they must first be introduced into a scavenging system. Once they have escaped from the anesthesia machine or breathing circuit, they must be removed by the operating room ventilation. It is poor practice to leave the anesthetic gases turned on while removing the mask from the face of the patient or disconnecting the breathing circuit. It also pays to be conscientious about leak checks of both the high- and low-pressure systems on the anesthesia machine in order to avoid contamination of room air.

A properly designed collection and scavenging system is also necessary. This consists of connections to the pop-off valves of the absorber and ventilator and a safety interface to protect against both positive- and negative-pressure buildup. Scavenging systems that depend on charcoal filters will work for the volatile agents but have little absorbing effect on nitrous oxide. Techniques of merely dumping the anesthetic near the floor are not effective in removing it from the operating room. The collected gases can be removed by exhaust into a nonrecirculating air conditioning return grill, a separate blower and duct system, or properly designed suction systems.

Following these recommendations, an effective scavenging system can be devised to remove the anesthetics from the operating room environment and to send them out of the hospital in a nonrecirculating exhaust system. However, just because they are now out of the hospital itself does not mean that they are no longer a problem. It must be determined that maintenance personnel or others are not routinely exposed to the waste gases at the point of exit from the hospital.

But, perhaps of more importance, we have not removed the waste anesthetic hazard. Rather, we have shifted it from one system to another. These waste anesthetics are no longer part of the system or environment that is defined by the four walls of the operating room; however, they now will reside for some period of time and have an effect in the atmosphere.

System Three: Atmospheric Effects of the Waste Anesthetics

The atmosphere itself can also be defined as a system. It is open to energy input from the sun and radiates energy back into space. Gases and other airborne substances circulate within the atmosphere or are exchanged between earth and sky. The waste anesthetic gases, owing to the same stability preventing toxic effects in the body, typically have a very long residence time within the atmosphere. Although they do not appear to have direct toxic effect on living species because of extremely low concentration in the atmosphere, they can participate in many chemical reactions that have an impact on life. The effects of primary interest fall under two general headings: the greenhouse effect and impact on the ozone production/destruction cycle. Though they have somewhat similar environmental effects, nitrous oxide and the volatile agents have differences in their mechanisms of action. Because of these differences, each will be examined separately.

NITROUS OXIDE IN THE ATMOSPHERE

Under conditions of normal temperature and pressure, and in the absence of excessive radiation, nitrous oxide is a relatively unreactive substance. Because it does not participate in chemical reactions under standard conditions, it does not decompose readily in the troposphere, that body of air lying next to the surface and extending to an altitude of approximately 6 miles. Although it is related to the other nitric compounds (NO_x), it does not contribute directly to acid rain. However, because it does not participate in chemical reactions in the troposphere, it resides in the atmosphere long enough to make its way to the stratosphere, 6 to 15 miles in altitude. Once there, nitrous oxide participates as a catalyst in ozone destruction. The overall nitrous oxide cycle is shown in Figure 2. Ultraviolet radiation in the stratosphere leads to a photolysis reaction which produces singlet oxygen. Singlet oxygen, when combined with nitrous oxide in the presence of ultraviolet radiation, leads to formation of two nitric oxide molecules. These nitric oxide molecules participate directly in the catalytic destruction of ozone until they, too, are combined with hydroxide ions to form nitric acid. This nitric acid leaves the stratosphere and falls back to earth.[14]

It would be misleading to say that this destruction cycle of ozone is not a natural occurrence. Indeed, the nitrous oxide produced for med-

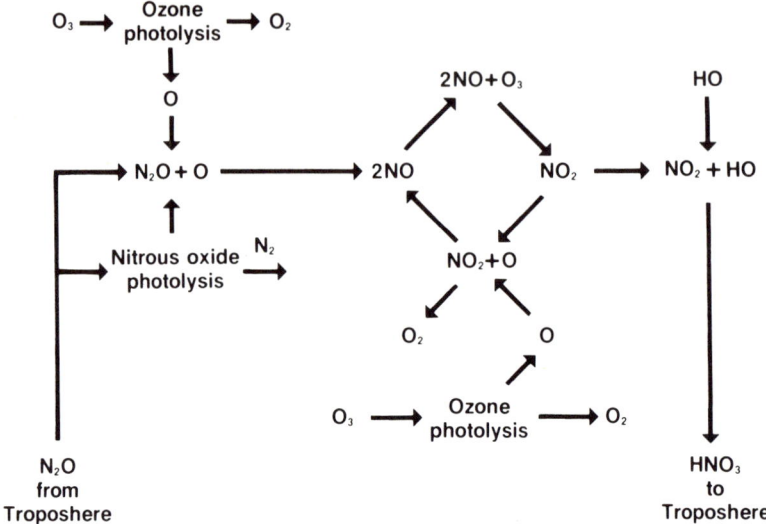

Figure 2. Role of nitrous oxide in ozone destruction and nitric acid production in stratosphere. (Adapted from *Nitrates: An Environmental Assessment.* National Academy Press, Washington, DC, 1978, with permission.)

ical purposes is a very small amount relative to that released to the atmosphere from other sources. The most significant of these other sources are nitrification in fertilizer production and natural processes of microorganisms in soil. Natural sinks for nitrous oxide other than the stratosphere also exist. Estimates of the balance of nitrous oxide from the sources and sinks add up to a net flux of nitrous oxide into the atmosphere ranging from 10 to 100 teragrams (1 teragram = 1 × 10^{12} grams) per year.[14,15] Exact figures on this nitrous oxide flux are not available. Similarly, exact figures on the use of nitrous oxide for medical purposes are not available. In Great Britain, it has been estimated that the use of nitrous oxide lies in the range of 4 to 40 liters per person per year.[16] Rough estimates of use in the United States are similar. If a use of 15 liters per capita is extrapolated to the worldwide population, the medical use of nitrous oxide would still count for much less than 1 percent of the total yearly flux (0.1 teragram worldwide medical use).

Because the medical use of nitrous oxide accounts for a relatively small proportion of its total atmospheric flux, it has been largely neglected in the literature on effects of nitrous oxide in the atmosphere. This is not to say, however, that its effect is going to be insignificant in the long run. Although it is not presently of overwhelming importance, it may have long-term effects owing to its long residence time and stability in the troposphere. Because ozone is constantly produced and destroyed in the atmosphere, the actual concentration is caused by a balance between these two processes. Any alteration in the rate of either of these processes could cause a significant long-term change in the end concentration. Also, because nitrous oxide absorbs radiation in the infrared spectrum, a possibility exists that it contributes to the so-called greenhouse effect. This effect is explored more fully in relation to the volatile anesthetics but may apply to nitrous oxide as well. At present, the production of fertilizer is of much greater concern because of its significantly greater impact upon nitrous oxide fluxes. However, a proper attitude for the medical profession might be the same one applied to the setting of exposure limits for waste anesthetics in the operating room: Reduce the release of nitrous oxide and volatile agents into the atmosphere to as low a level as practical.

ATMOSPHERIC EFFECTS OF THE HALOGENATED AGENTS

The volatile anesthetic agents are not as stable as nitrous oxide within the troposphere. Halothane most likely breaks down very readily when exposed to ultraviolet radiation. However, as the search for potent agents that do not produce toxic metabolic substances in the body has progressed, more stable compounds have been introduced. These compounds should also have longer residence times in the atmosphere. Because of this, the tropospheric and stratospheric effects should be considered. At present, volatile anesthetic agents have not been fully examined for environmental effects. However, because of their similarities to other halogenated hydrocarbons, some inferences may be made about the possible atmospheric impact. The two effects of concern are the greenhouse effect and ozone destruction.

The first of these effects, the greenhouse effect, relates to a rise in global surface temperature because substances in the atmosphere absorb infrared radiation and then radiate heat. Chlorofluorocarbons as a group contain infrared spectral absorption bands in the region of 8 to 13 μm. At this wavelength the atmosphere is relatively transparent. Because of this transparency, radiation in this band would not otherwise be absorbed and would not cause heat to be released to produce a temperature rise. However, when substances such as the chlorofluorocarbons are present to absorb this energy, atmospheric temperature is raised, which in turn radiates heat to the earth's surface.[17] The global effects of an atmospheric temperature rise are still somewhat controversial. However, it is probably undesirable for animal life to be subjected to an experiment to find out what these effects may be. Again, the medical use of anesthetic agents is not the major culprit. There are several fluorocarbon compounds produced and released into the atmosphere for other purposes, including the well-known freons. Also, volatile anesthetic agents have not been exclusively studied nor has any mass balance been attempted to assess the significance of halogenated anesthetic agents in relationship to the greenhouse effect. However, once more reason suggests that it would be most desirable to prevent release of these substances to the atmosphere if possible.

A second possible effect of halogenated agents is the contribution to ozone destruction in the stratosphere.[18,19] If they are able to survive in the troposphere for the several years necessary to reach the stratosphere, it is conceivable that they might undergo photolysis. This breakdown can release chloride and fluoride ions. Released ions would again participate in the ozone depletion cycle. However, because such atmospheric chemistry has not been extensively studied, it is not known whether the halogenated anesthetic agents possess adequate stability to survive in the troposphere long enough to reach the stratosphere. If survival is long enough, impact on ozone destruction needs to be assessed.

Although waste anesthetic agents are not of primary concern to atmospheric scientists because of the relatively small quantities released, they may have been unduly neglected. Perhaps it is time to study their environmental effects and explore ways of reducing the ecologic impact. The simplest solution seems to be that of reducing the release as much as possible. This would limit the environmental impact and possibly could provide other benefits.

A PROPOSED PROCESS FOR RECOVERY AND RECYCLING OF WASTE ANESTHETIC AND RESPIRATORY GASES

Having argued against the release of exhaled and overflow gases into the operating room or atmosphere, some corrective scheme must be developed. One such proposal is to accumulate the expired and waste gases, separate the mixture into useful components, and then reuse or discard the components as appropriate. Methods other than the one outlined below may be possible, and other ways of dealing with the problem could offer greater advantage. However, estimates of feasibility, cost, and benefits can be made for the proposed process.

The system that is proposed for recovery and recycling of the anesthetic and respiratory gases is shown in Figure 3. This system is presently only a hypothetical concept, but each component within it is either an established technique or a process used in similar industrial or experimental situations.

The first part of the system is an active scavenging system to recover the gases escaping from the breathing circle or ventilator pop-off valve. The interfaces currently available are suitable for this application without modification. The gases expected at this point are oxygen, carbon dioxide, water vapor, nitrous oxide, and volatile anesthetic vapor.

The next device is an absorber to remove the carbon dioxide. This can be the same chemical absorbent currently in use but must be examined for possible degradation of either absorbent or anesthetic agent. After this step, the gas mixture consists of water vapor, oxygen, nitrous oxide, and volatile agent.

The third step is removal of water vapor either by a desiccant or by mechanical means, such as a trap and vortex tube. This leaves only oxygen, nitrous oxide, and volatile agent. The second and third steps may be transposed in practice if this is indicated to prevent the degradation previously mentioned.

Volatile anesthetic is removed next by cooling the gas mixture. While nitrous oxide also will condense at low temperatures ($-88.6°C$ at 1 atmosphere), adequate recovery of the volatile agent in this distillation process is possible at temperatures that will avoid this problem. For instance, at $-80°C$, isoflurane has a vapor pressure of 0.27 mm Hg. This corresponds to a concentration of 0.036 percent. If an inspiratory concentration of 2 percent is used, the recovery efficiency is 98 percent. The recovered liquid agent can be collected and returned to the vaporizer for reuse. This would cut ultimate consumption to about 2 percent of its former level.

After the volatile agent is removed, the remaining gas is a mixture of oxygen and nitrous oxide. Unfortunately it cannot be used directly because of variable concentration. However, by compressing the mixture, nitrous oxide will liquefy and can then be separated from the oxygen. These two components can then be stored for reuse.

The first three steps need to be performed on a per machine basis because each location may use a specific volatile agent. The final step can be done in a central location.

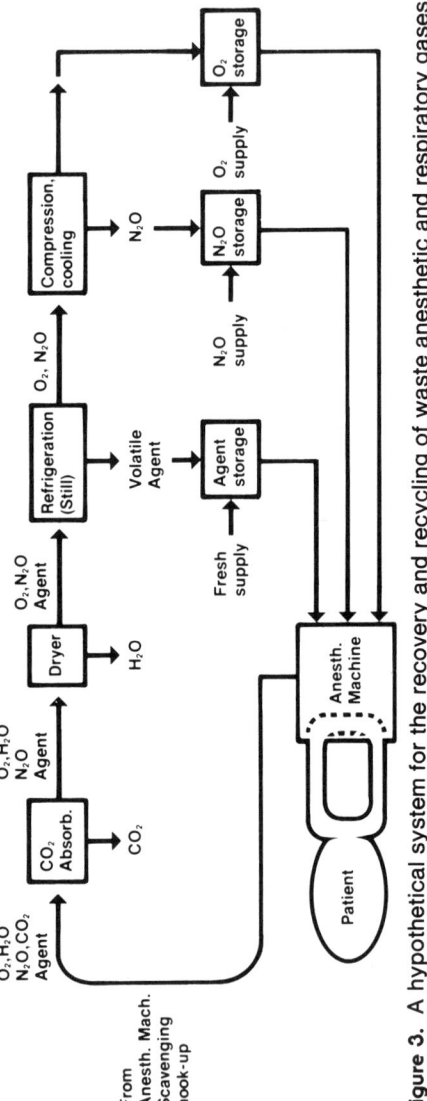

Figure 3. A hypothetical system for the recovery and recycling of waste anesthetic and respiratory gases.

Obviously many questions arise from the proposed scheme. Can the components of the gas mixture be recovered in suitable quality and purity for reuse? When impurities are the same components added for inhalation use, what purity level is acceptable? Are the benefits derived from such a process sufficient to warrant its implementation? An estimate can be made of the potential costs and benefits, but these other questions must be addressed before overall feasibility can be assessed.

Cost-Benefit Analysis

As with all proposed changes, there are certain costs associated with not changing and other expenses in making a change. In the case of recovering waste anesthetics, the benefits and costs are not well defined owing to inexperience in addressing the problem. However, there are some expenses that one can logically suppose will be associated with recovering the waste anesthetics. These costs fall into the categories of energy and equipment. To assess the possible expenditures necessary, let us consider a hypothetical example.

For example,* let us assume we have an operating suite of eight rooms handling 5500 cases a year, the majority of which are general anesthetics using inhalation agents. One such hospital may use as much as 4 metric tons of nitrous oxide in a year. The yearly use of volatile agents could be expected to be about 112 liters, divided unevenly amongst the three most commonly used drugs: halothane, enflurane, and isoflurane.

Using a recovery scheme such as that outlined, the energy expenditure to compress and to liquefy this amount of nitrous oxide approaches $700 (assuming 3 cents per kilowatt-hour electricity). This is (we hope) a worst-case cost estimate based on less than 25 percent efficiency in compression and cooling processes. This $700 energy cost is in comparison to the $8000 it would cost to purchase 4 metric tons of nitrous oxide. Obviously, some capital equipment must be purchased and maintained, but if capital maintenance and quality assurance costs total less than $7300, the hospital will save money by recycling nitrous oxide. At present the assumption of a cost figure for equipment and operation cannot be objectively evaluated because pilot plant data are unavailable. However, it seems reason-

---

*Case loads and drug usage figures are based on actual data from a 300+ bed tertiary-care teaching hospital.

able that the necessary equipment would have a long life span and should cost considerably less than $6000 per year.

The potential for savings on volatile agents is even greater. Although the equipment necessary to recover and to redistribute these agents would undoubtedly be more expensive than that necessary for nitrous oxide, these potent anesthetics are also considerably more expensive. Expenditures for our hypothetical institution could be expected to total $40,000 per year for halothane, enflurane, and isoflurane. Energy costs for recovery should be approximately $1,000, leaving a significant portion for equipment expenses.

Although the most readily quantifiable benefits are fiscal, recovery and recycling would be accompanied by environmental benefits as well. Although medical use accounts for only a small portion of the fluorocarbons and nitrous oxide released into the atmosphere, a responsibility exists to reduce these sources as much as possible.

SUMMARY

The problem of waste anesthetic gases must be addressed because of potential health hazards. However, solutions must be considered within a larger context than that of the operating room or dental suite. The impact of shifting wastes from the hospital into the atmosphere must be examined for both ecologic and ethical implications. A hypothetic situation has been proposed in which the waste anesthetics are dealt with by recovery and reuse. Although potential costs and benefits can be discussed, overall feasibility and desirability cannot be assessed until certain questions are addressed. Are waste anesthetic gases an atmospheric pollutant with impact sufficient to cause concern? If not, do the economic considerations of recycling exhausted anesthetic and respiratory gases warrant implementation? Anesthesiologists need to consider these issues within the constraints of the environments in which they practice. The problem will exist as long as inhalation anesthesia is in use. Solution should not create new problems.

REFERENCES

1. ASA Ad Hoc Committee: *Occupational disease among operating room personnel: A national study.* Anesthesiology 41:321–340, 1974.

2. COHEN, EN: *Toxicity of inhalation anaesthetic agents.* Br J Anaesth 50:665, 1978.
3. COATE, WB, KAPP, RW, LEWIS, TR: *Chronic exposure to low concentration of halothane-nitrous oxide: Reproductive and cytogenetic effects in the rat.* Anesthesiology 50:310–318, 1979.
4. *Criteria for recommended standard-occupational exposure to waste anesthetic gases and vapors.* HEW Publication No. (NIOSH) 77-140. US Department of Health, Education, and Welfare, 1977.
5. FINK, BR AND CULLEN, BF: *Anesthetic pollution: What is happening to us?* Anesthesiology 45:79–83, 1976.
6. FERSTANDIG, LL: *Trace concentration of anesthetic gases: A critical review of their disease potential.* Anesth Analg 57:328–345, 1978.
7. MILLER, MG AND CULLEN, BF: *The cost of scavenging—is it worth it?* Anesth Analg 58:265–266, 1979.
8. WOOD, M, O'MALLEY, K, STEVENSON, IH: *Drug metabolizing ability in operating theatre personnel.* Br J Anaesth 46:726–728, 1974.
9. WHITCHER, C, ET AL: *Development and evaluation of methods for the elimination of waste anesthetic gases and vapors in hospitals.* HEW Publication No. (NIOSH) 75-137. US Department of Health, Education, and Welfare, 1975.
10. MCINTYRE, JWR, PURDHAM, JT, HOSEIN, HR. *An assessment of operating room environment air contamination with nitrous oxide and halothane and some scavenging methods.* Canad Anaesth Soc J 25:499, 1978.
11. SASS-KORTSAK, AM, WHEELER, IP, PURDHAM, JT: *Exposure of operating room personnel to anaesthetic agents: An examination of the effectiveness of scavenging systems and the importance of maintenance programs.* Canad Anaesth Soc J 28:22–28, 1981.
12. TORDA, TA, JONES, R, ENGLERT, J: *A study of waste gas scavenging in operating theatres.* Anaesth Intens Care 6:215–221, 1978.
13. THOMPSON, JM, ET AL: *Evaluation of the efficacy of an active scavenger for controlling air contamination in an operating theatre.* Br J Anaesth 53:235–240, 1981.
14. NATIONAL ACADEMY OF SCIENCES PANEL ON NITRATES: *Nitrates: An Environmental Assessment.* National Academy Press, Washington, DC, 1978.
15. DELWICH, CC (ED): *Denitrification, Nitrification, and Atmospheric Nitrous Oxide.* John Wiley & Sons, New York, 1981.
16. GRANT, WJ: *Medical Gases: Their Properties and Uses.* Year Book Medical Publishers, Chicago, 1978.
17. RAMANATHAN, V: *Greenhouse effect due to chlorofluorocarbons: Climactic implications.* Science 190:50–52, 1975.

18. NATIONAL ACADEMY OF SCIENCES PANEL ON LOW MOLECULAR WEIGHT HALOGENATED HYDROCARBONS: *Chloroform, Carbon Tetrachloride, and Other Halomethanes: An Environmental Assessment.* National Academy Press, Washington, DC, 1978.
19. NATIONAL ACADEMY OF SCIENCES PANEL ON STRATOSPHERIC CHEMISTRY AND TRANSPORT: *Stratospheric Ozone Depletion by Halocarbone: Chemistry and Transport.* National Academy Press, Washington, DC, 1979.

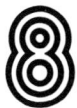

CONTROL OF ANESTHETIC DELIVERY

Kenneth C. Mylrea, Ph.D.

This chapter provides a basic description of control system theory as it applies to anesthesia delivery. Control can be described as a means of guiding or regulating the operation of a machine, apparatus, or system. Implementing control requires that there be a desirable behavior and a means of predictably altering that behavior. Also, we must be able to measure some behavioral characteristic(s) to determine whether or not the system is operating as desired.

The first recorded control systems appeared about 250 BC when a float regulator was used to maintain the level of oil in a lamp.[1] In modern Europe the first control systems with feedback for temperature and pressure regulation appeared in the 16th and 17th centuries.[2] Feedback is the term used when information concerning the behavior of the system (output) is fed back to modify the operation of the system (usually at the input). Although control systems can operate with or without feedback, systems with feedback (closed loop) have many beneficial characteristics.

Most theory and applications of control systems evolved in response to needs in telephone system development, autopilots, gun positioning and radar control in World War II and in missile control and satellite guidance during the space age.[2] Automatic control theory has now advanced to the point where multiple-variable systems can be analyzed and constructed for optimal control of one or more characteristics. Our concern here is to what extent these theories and knowledge can be applied to the problems and requirements surrounding anesthesia delivery in the operating room.

The very process of anesthesia delivery is a control system with a human providing the feedback, i.e., an attempt to control anesthetic concentration in the brain. The anesthetic overrides or modifies other physiologic systems, e.g., respiratory and cardiovascular systems. Thus, there are two aspects of control in anesthesia delivery: monitoring and control of the delivery of a predetermined amount or concentration of anesthetic to the patient and monitoring and control of physiologic variables.

We will use the term *variable* for an output characteristic (measurement) of a system and the term *parameter* for a characteristic that we change or set at a desired value. These terms allow a more generalized description of a system with characteristics (variables) we want to control and characteristics (parameters) we can change to effect that control. The same characteristic can be a variable in some situations and a parameter in others. For example, we can adjust anesthetic concentration (a parameter) in response to changes in blood pressure (a variable), or we can adjust a blood pressure (a parameter) to control fluid volumes, cardiac output, and so forth.

Physiologic systems are normally self-controlling, complex, and highly interactive. Self-controlling implies an internal feedback such that the physiologic system works to maintain the value of its variables. Because of the interdependence of physiologic systems, the corrective action for controlling a patient variable may depend on the status of several other variables. For these reasons, incorporating physiologic variables into a control system can significantly increase the complexity.

Control systems that involve only technology are less complex and more predictable. An example of such a system is the control of inspired gases. A system can be based on technology but encompass a physiologic variable, e.g., control of end-tidal anesthetic concentration by adjusting inspired concentration. Such systems may require two modes of operation. The control system would function as designed as long as other variables (e.g., blood pressure, respiration) are within prescribed ranges; otherwise an alarm would alert the attendant to appraise the situation for possible corrective action. This combination system is an appropriate mechanism for introducing control systems and may remain the standard mode of action in clinical applications.

WHAT IS A CONTROL SYSTEM?

Although theoretical analysis and application of control systems can be complex, it is not difficult to obtain a conceptual understanding of the process and the potential benefits. This section provides only a brief introduction to the concepts. The interested reader is encouraged to pursue the subject through available texts.[2,3]

A control system can be described as the interconnection of components to form a system that will bring about a desired response. There are two basic types of control systems: open loop and closed loop (Fig. 1). An open loop system allows the operator to set an input parameter such that the desired output will be obtained under normal circumstances. An example is the automobile accelerator which can be set to produce a desired speed on a level highway. However, as the vehicle moves uphill or downhill the speed will change because, without human intervention, there is no correction of the accelerator

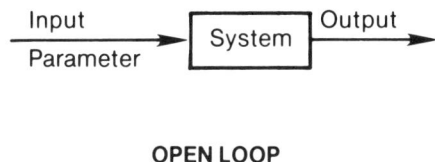

OPEN LOOP

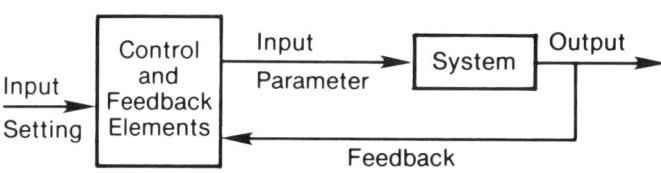

CLOSED LOOP

Figure 1. Two basic types of control systems are *(top)* open loop and *(bottom)* closed loop.

position. Thus, in the open loop system, if the circumstances change, the system output moves away from the desired value.

A closed loop control system automatically changes an input parameter to maintain the desired output. The automobile cruise control does this by automatically adjusting accelerator position to maintain the desired speed. A predetermined corrective response is automatically activated when the output changes from the desired value. A closed loop system incorporates feedback by sensing and evaluating the output variable and feeding information back to the input for appropriate corrective action.

Feedback produces several beneficial features. It can allow the system to respond only to certain types of change in the output, e.g., the cruise control does not respond to a bumpy road but does respond to slower changes in speed. Additionally, feedback can make a system more stable, can reduce the sensitivity to changes in temperature or environment, and can reduce the effect of external disturbances (noise) on the system. Corrective action can be an on-off response (like a home thermostat), a function of the difference between desired and actual output, the summation of the difference seen over time, or some combination of these.

Control systems can become unstable if the corrective action is applied without consideration of time delays. If the system responds slowly to corrective action, a delay in the rate of correction is needed to avoid overcompensation. Inherent delays can exist in various parts of a system such as sensor, correcting mechanism, or system response. Normally it is desirable to have as fast a response as possible without overcorrection or oscillation. Extensive theory has been developed to analyze systems for stability. For interactive, physiologic systems, common sense and experience may prove to be an equally useful approach.

Control systems can be linear or nonlinear, time invariant or time varying, continuous or sampled. These complexities need not concern us here, except to note the additional capability which is available through the use of microprocessors and microcomputers as part of a control system. Computers require data sampling, i.e., the variables are measured at periodic intervals rather than continuously monitored. However, the rate at which measurements are made (sampling rates) can be sufficiently high so that the signals appear to be continuously monitored. Microprocessors can be self-checking (to determine whether the instrument is operating correctly), and they allow decision-making algorithms to be part of the control system. Thus, the type and amount of corrective action can be complex functions of many different variables measured frequently and concurrently. The functions are similar to those an anesthesiologist performs, but faster and without fatigue or inattention.

Control is different from monitoring. A monitor can exist without control, but a closed loop control system cannot exist without monitoring. A monitor measures one or more variables and provides information (and perhaps a warning) when certain prescribed conditions are not met. The closed loop control system takes action to correct the undesirable conditions. This brings up an interesting point: Can a human be a part of the closed loop control system? This is, in fact, the situation, for humans respond to monitor alarms and apply corrective action to the measured variables. The question itself may be moot, but it allows us to consider the concept of complex decision making as part of a closed loop control system. The anesthesiologist takes in information about one or more variables, integrates this information with data from the "memory bank," and effects some response. The real question is whether or not the decision-making process can be automated and the responses uniquely defined. This concept will be explored in detail later in this chapter.

CONTROLLING PHYSIOLOGIC VARIABLES

Control systems are well known in the technologic world. For instance, a rocket is sent away from earth and guided to a soft landing at a specific site on the moon while maintaining its internal environment. This activity involves extensive use of feedback control systems, with many input parameters and multiple outputs. Why is it so difficult to apply this technology to physiologic problems? Probably the primary reason is that the system in question, the human, is a complex set of interdependent, multiparameter, nonlinear closed loop control systems. Additionally, we do not totally understand some of these control systems and are probably not even aware of others. $PaCO_2$, PaO_2, pH, respiration, blood volume, and other variables all operate with their own control systems and yet are interdependent. Thus, although technical theories can provide useful inputs, we must be aware that the physiologic system is a highly controlled, potentially unstable system with both conscious and subconscious, evident and hidden, controllers.

The situation is further complicated in the anesthetized patient with a few normal control systems partially or totally inoperative. Respiration may be turned off completely and blood pressure control present but modified. We already have devices to control respiration, but these involve primarily open loop control. Respirator parameters are adjusted by a human operator if and when physiologic variables need to be changed. To control blood pressure we must cope with a partially functioning physiologic control system. Furthermore, the responses of the patient's blood pressure provide information regarding the depth of anesthesia, and we would like to retain this source of information and not just maintain a constant pressure.

There are physiologic variables we would like to control, such as $PaCO_2$, PaO_2, anesthetic concentration, blood pressure, and heart rate; and there are input parameters we can adjust, e.g., respiration depth and rate, oxygen and anesthetic concentration, and drug infusion. The interactive nature of these variables and parameters contraindicates a simple single-variable control system. For example, it may not be wise to control anesthetic concentration based on blood pressure alone. However, we may be able to monitor several variables and automatically adjust one or more parameters to control a particular characteristic throughout a variety of patient circumstances. For such conditions, a computer with memory and complex decision-making capability will be an indispensable tool.

WHAT CAN BE CONTROLLED IN ANESTHESIA DELIVERY

Controlling the status of a system is a natural extension of monitoring, about which an extensive review regarding anesthesia is available.[4] Monitoring is currently undertaken to provide information about a system or to obtain the value of a variable that must be maintained within certain limits. Both functions may be carried out simultaneously. For example, blood pressure is monitored as one indication of depth of anesthesia; however, corrective action is taken should the pressure wander outside reasonable limits. To control a variable, we must know its numerical value and have sufficient experience to predict changes in response to intentional interventions or ancillary events. Thus, appropriate applications of control systems in anesthesia delivery will be found in situations where a variable is monitored and its value predictably maintained by human intervention. Automating the human intervention creates a closed loop control system.

We have discussed the difference between controlling equipment variables and controlling patient variables. Equipment control is more predictable and involves monitoring and control of the instruments and devices around the patient, e.g., the control of oxygen concentration in the anesthesia circuit. Most anesthesia delivery systems now have the potential for monitoring oxygen concentration. Automatic control of this variable can be accomplished with a valve on the oxygen supply, automatically adjusted to provide the desired concentration of oxygen in the circuit. In flow-through (high-flow) anesthesia delivery, the response is predictable and easily automated. In a closed-circuit system, complications arise because of the interdependence on volumes and absorption rates of other gases, but the response is still predictable. A closed loop control system to control oxygen concentration and circuit volume in a closed-circuit system has been used in several hundred surgical cases.[5] The system controls circuit volume by nitrous oxide (N_2O) flow and controls inspired oxygen concentration via oxygen flow. It is interesting to note that this system has the potential for an unstable or oscillating response without appropriate delays in the corrective actions.

Flow adjustments on anesthesia machines are examples of open loop control systems. Flow is measured via rotameters, but there is no automatic correction if any of the flows change. Because rotameter inaccuracies can be from 20 to 50 percent,[6] closed loop control of gas concentrations from anesthesia equipment would be useful. This would maintain preset concentrations of oxygen, nitrous oxide, and anesthetic in the breathing circuit. Keeping in mind that a control system requires a monitoring capability, the lack of reliable, accurate, and inexpensive sensors for different gases may be the reason such systems are not yet available.[7]

Control of physiologic variables is still in the investigative stages but has been accomplished in the postoperative cardiac surgical patient.[8] A computer operating in a closed loop control system monitors heart rate, intra-arterial pressure, right and left atrial pressure, rectal temperature, chest tube drainage, and urine output. Infusion of blood or albumin and of vasoactive agents is automatically controlled using decision-making algorithms involving stroke volume, left atrial pressure, and mean pressure. Several attempts at closed loop control of arterial carbon dioxide via changes in ventilation have been attempted, with the primary problems related to accurate and reliable sampling of the variables.[9] The above work indicates both the feasibility and the difficulties of control for physiologic variables. In anesthesia, an appropriate starting point for closed loop automatic control may be the gas delivery system, with which fewer problems can be expected.

Physiologic theory and empirical studies in anesthesia delivery[10,11] point out a few of the conditions and trends that may be useful in introducing control systems. End-tidal anesthetic concentration gives an indication of arterial levels and can be used as one of the measured variables in a control system. Although this is a physiologic variable, it is not actively controlled by the body and thus is not subject to the caveats of self-controlling physiologic variables. Additionally, we can automatically control inspired anesthetic concentration to bring about the desired blood level in the shortest time. In animal experiments an anesthetic monitor with a microprocessor was used in a closed-circuit system to determine the amount and time of liquid anesthetic injection into the circle.[12] The anesthetic monitor[13] was not fast enough to discriminate end-tidal values, so average inspired anesthetic concentration was the controlled variable.

The potential of closed loop control systems in anesthesia delivery can be seen through the experimental situation depicted in Figure 2.

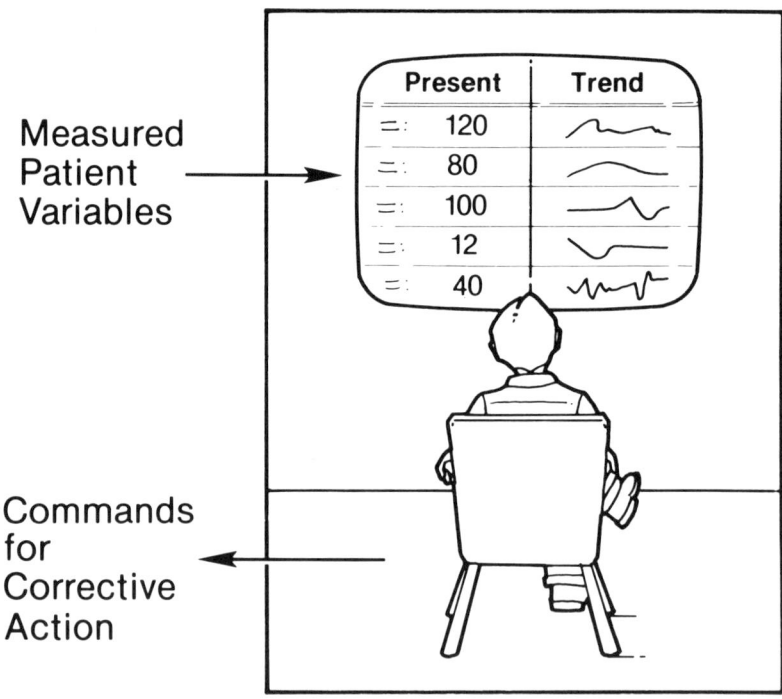

Figure 2. An important feature for control of anesthesia delivery is observation of measured patient variables and subsequent commands for corrective action by the anesthesiologist.

An anesthesiologist sits outside the operating room viewing a display of the patient's physiologic variables. Only information that can be automatically measured is presented, although one could use trends or past values. If there are definable and predictable responses for patient management, these maintenance actions could be delegated to an automatic system. The question may also be characterized as a determination of whether or not the use of the existing knowledge base and inference mechanisms can be defined as an algorithm.[14] Although this example may illustrate a point, it is not intended to indicate that closed loop control systems can remove the anesthetist from the patient setting. In fact, one of the goals is to allow the individual more time to deal directly with the patient. The analogy between anesthesiologists and airline pilots holds here. Automatic control systems allow the pilot more opportunity to use personal background, training, and intuition to manage the situation, rather than just to direct the airplane.

BENEFITS FROM AUTOMATIC CONTROL SYSTEMS IN ANESTHESIA

Automatic control systems can reduce the tedium of routine activities. This relief from routine activities is similar to that obtained with automobile cruise control. The driver presets a speed with assurance that this speed will be automatically maintained. The driver can then focus attention on driving, potential hazards, or conversation in the car.

Another benefit is the reduced requirement for continuous vigilance. Because it is physically impossible to maintain vigilance for extended periods, the assistance of a system to maintain control in routine situations and to provide alarms when appropriate should be welcomed. Understandably, vigilance is still the anesthesiologist's responsibility. The system is an aid, not a substitute, for a skilled physician.

Additional cost can be expected from the increase in technology. However, there may be savings as well. Closed-circuit anesthesia systems produce significant savings from the decrease in anesthetic agents used.

Benefits from control systems in anesthesia might best be viewed as potential reductions in morbidity and mortality. Studies of critical incidents in anesthesia delivery[15] indicate that measurable improvements are certainly possible. Another way to envision benefits is to imagine that you are a patient in an average hospital with an average anesthetist. Which of your variables would you like to have under automatic control, assuming the control system can be made reliable and effective? The cost/benefit ratio can be assessed only after the technology is developed; we must proceed on reasonable expectations, rather than hard data.

FUTURE DIRECTIONS IN ANESTHESIA CONTROL

In medicine, new monitoring techniques are often delayed because the need for another measurement has not been established. Without the need there is little incentive to develop the capability. An example of this is an anesthetic concentration monitor. If such a device were currently available, it might not be used because the anesthetist does not know what to do with the numbers and because benefits have not yet been demonstrated. On the other hand, the benefits from monitoring and/or control of anesthetic concentration cannot be demonstrated until such a measurement is possible.

Control systems in anesthesia delivery will require new or improved measurements and monitoring techniques. Considerable work is underway to quantitate the depth of anesthesia through electroencephalogram analysis. Only after an acceptable technique is available can systems be developed to control anesthetic concentrations to maintain the desired depth of anesthesia. A control system for oxygen concentration and the maintenance of volume in closed-circuit anesthesia has already been mentioned.[5] In addition to this, algorithms are being developed that use respiratory flow and expired gas concentrations to derive breath-by-breath data, trend analysis, and cumulative information regarding a patient's anesthetic status.[16] Other investigations are underway to quantitate neuromuscular block and differentiate the type and phase of block present.[17,18]

In the above attempts to monitor and to control physiologic variables, the primary obstacle is the lack of reliable, rugged, and inexpensive sensors. Thus, research in control systems for anesthesia must include development of sensors and transducers to measure reliably the variables in question. Also, continuing research is needed to determine which variables to control and the appropriate algorithms to effect control.

REFERENCES

1. MAYR, O: *The origins of feedback control.* Sci Am 223:4, pp. 110–118, October, 1970.
2. DORF, RC: *Modern Control Systems.* Addison-Wesley, Reading, MA, 1980.

3. Kuo, BC: *Automatic Control Systems.* Prentice-Hall, Englewood Cliffs, NJ, 1982.
4. Saidman, LJ and Smith, NT: *Monitoring in Anesthesia.* John Wiley & Sons, New York, 1978.
5. Westenskow, DR, Jordan, WS, Hayes, JK: *Closed-loop control of the closed circuit anesthesia breathing circuit.* Proceedings AAMI 17th Annual Meeting, May, 1982.
6. Saunders, RJ, Calkins, JM, Gooden, TG: *Accuracy of rotameters and linear flowmeters.* Anesthesiology (Supp) 55:A116, 1981.
7. Mylrea, KC, et al: *Automated anesthesia delivery and patient management in the operating room.* In Karni, S (ed): *24th Midwest Symposium on Circuits and Systems.* Univ of New Mexico Press, 1981, pp 667–673.
8. Sheppard, LC and Kouchoukas, NT: *Management of the postoperative cardiac surgical patient.* In Rackley, C (ed): *Critical Care Cardiology.* Cardiovascular Clinics Series, vol 11, number 3. FA Davis, Philadelphia, 1981, pp 131–139.
9. Westenskow, DR: *Control of $PaCO_2$ during mechanical ventilation: Monitoring and feedback techniques.* Annals of Biomedical Engineering, vol 9, number 5-6, p. 659, 1981.
10. Eger, EI, II: *Anesthetic Uptake and Action.* Williams & Wilkins, Baltimore, 1978.
11. Lowe, HJ and Ernst, EA: *The Quantitative Practice of Anesthesia, Use of Closed Circuit.* Williams & Wilkins, Baltimore, 1981.
12. Mylrea, KC, et al: *Closed loop anesthesia delivery under microprocessor control.* Proceedings AAMI 15th Annual Meeting, 1980.
13. Calkins, JM, et al: *A new electromechanical anesthetic monitor.* 1980 Frontiers of Engineering in Health Care, IEEE, Piscataway, NJ, 1980, pp 101–104.
14. Reggia, JA: *Computer-assisted medical decision making: A critical review.* Annals of Biomedical Engineering, vol 9, number 5-6, 1981, p 605.
15. Cooper, JB et al: *Preventable anesthesia mishaps: A study of human factors.* Anesthesiology 49:399, 1978.
16. Lauria, MJ, et al: *A real time data acquisition and processing system.* 1982 Frontiers of Engineering in Health Care, IEEE, Piscataway, NJ, 1982, p 288.
17. Ham, RE, Mylrea, KC, Adler, L: *Integration of muscular response—a new method of measuring neuromuscular blockade.* Proceedings AAMI 14th Annual Meeting, May, 1979.
18. Fiore, MD, et al: *A microprocessor-based neuromuscular blockade monitor.* IEEE Transactions on Biomedical Engineering, vol BME-28, 1981, p 775.

MONITORING SYSTEM GAS CONCENTRATIONS
Jerry M. Calkins, Ph.D., M.D.

Recent advances in technology for gas analysis have made new instruments commercially available to anesthesiologists. Some reasonable questions now are being asked:

"Why do we need to monitor gases in the first place?"

"These measurements have not been routine in the past!"

"What kind of useful information are these numbers going to yield?"

"Anesthesiologists already have too much to worry about!"

"There are too many gadgets now!"

We believe that the anesthesiologist needs to monitor the anesthetic and respiratory gases found within the machine and circuit for three basic reasons: vigilance, control of depth of anesthesia, and physiologic assessment (Table 1).

Vigilance monitoring can assist in the prevention of critical incidents (disasters) by providing information about machine performance and

Table 1. Why Monitor Circuit Gases?

1. Vigilance monitoring
   a. Detection of sudden disruptions
   b. Detection of gradual changes
2. Control of depth of anesthesia
3. Determination of physiologic variables
   a. Cardiovascular function
   b. Respiratory function

patient status. The anesthetist can be alerted by vigilance monitors to gradual, insidious changes and also to sudden, catastrophic disruptions in gas conditions. The depth of anesthesia may more easily be controlled by precise measurement of anesthetic gas concentrations, particularly during exhalation. With accurate determination of circuit gas concentrations, various physiologic variables indicating the functional status of the cardiovascular and respiratory systems are easily obtained by simple calculations.

In any anesthesia delivery system, the gases flowing within the inhaled and exhaled circuit are easily accessible for analysis. These may be analyzed for the average concentration of gas constituents in the circuit in order to determine what is supplied to the patient and what is unused by the patient. In addition, estimates of in vivo blood levels can be made from the patient's end-tidal exhaled gas concentrations. From these values much information about the patient's entire anesthetic experience can be obtained by considering what goes in and what comes out.

GASES TO MONITOR

Theoretically, any gas contained in either the circuit or the patient can be analyzed. However, with today's technology, it may not be possible to routinely analyze all gases. However, because of usefulness, concentrations of oxygen, carbon dioxide, nitrous oxide, and the volatile anesthetic agents (halothane, enflurane, and isoflurane) should be monitored. The analysis of each offers information to aid in vigilance monitoring, to control depth of anesthesia, and to obtain physiologic information.

VIGILANCE MONITORING

Vigilance monitoring is the key to preventing critical incidents. It enables the anesthesiologist to determine both machine performance and patient status. By monitoring each gas, different pieces of information can be collected and the complete operational condition assessed.

For example, let us consider oxygen (Table 2). There are a variety of techniques determining oxygen concentrations commercially available. Monitoring oxygen for vigilance can safeguard adequate machine performance. Is the anesthesia machine delivering the gases at the desired concentrations? With proper oxygen vigilance monitoring, the potential disaster of reversing nitrous oxide and oxygen supply lines can be avoided. Is the oxygen concentration adequate and appropriate for each case? We can answer the question affirmatively

Table 2. Elements of Vigilance Monitoring

1. Oxygen
    a. Machine performance
        (1) Adequate oxygen concentration
    b. Patient
        (1) Prevention of inadequate oxygen
        (2) Content in inspired gas mixtures
2. Carbon dioxide
    a. Machine performance
        (1) Efficiency of CO_2 absorber
        (2) Adequate flows to prevent rebreathing (Bain, Jackson-Rees, and so forth)
    b. Patient
        (1) Adequate ventilation (respiration rate)
        (2) Embolization detection
        (3) Malignant hyperthermia
3. Nitrous oxide, volatile anesthetics
    a. Machine performance
        (1) Appropriate circuit concentrations
        (2) Appropriate agent
        (3) System leakage to environment
    b. Patient
        (1) Overdose prevention
        (2) Rate of uptake alarms

with proper gas monitoring. Vigilance oxygen monitoring will prevent an inadequate oxygen concentration and will provide information about the content of the inspired gas mixture. Of course, 40 or 50 percent oxygen in the anesthesia circuit does not mean that a particular patient is not hypoxic, because there are other factors besides the inspired oxygen concentration.

The analysis of carbon dioxide (capnography) also is easily accomplished and provides additional valuable information (see Table 2). For vigilance monitoring, machine performance information—including proper functioning of the carbon dioxide absorber, adequate flows to prevent rebreathing (particularly in rebreathing circuits), and adequate functioning of the breathing valves—is easily obtained. In addition, for the patient breathing spontaneously or requiring controlled ventilation, the appropriateness of minute ventilation can be assessed.

Changes in a patient's end-tidal carbon dioxide levels (which are at equilibrium with alveolar capillaries) might indicate significant status modifications. It has been well documented that end-tidal carbon dioxide decreases dramatically when air embolism occurs. Also, one of the first signals of malignant hyperthermia is an immediate increased production of carbon dioxide, which should be reflected in an increase in the end-tidal carbon dioxide concentration.

Monitoring of anesthetic gases (nitrous oxide, halothane, enflurane, and isoflurane) falls into a pattern similar to that of oxygen and carbon dioxide (see Table 2). By knowing the concentration of the volatile agents, vigilance over machine performance, both for appropriate circuit concentration and for correct agent, can be quickly and readily accomplished. In closed-circuit or low-flow anesthesia, proper gas monitoring can determine leakage to the environment.

DEPTH OF ANESTHESIA

Measurements of gas concentrations cannot determine directly the depth of anesthesia. However, by knowing concentrations with respect to other variables, such as respiration, depth can be inferred (Table 3).

From the concentration of oxygen, control of depth of anesthesia also can be aided because the quantity of nitrous oxide can be estimated. For patients breathing spontaneously, the respiratory pattern, rates of ventilation, and exhaled carbon dioxide concentrations will assist in controlling depth of anesthesia. Measurement of anesthetic

Table 3. Control of Depth of Anesthesia

1. Oxygen
    a. Estimate of nitrous oxide concentration
2. Carbon dioxide
    a. Respiration rate
        (1) ($PaCO_2$, ventilation response)
    b. Respiratory pattern
3. Nitrous oxide, volatile anesthetic agents
    a. Appropriate uptake rate (F_A/F_I)
        (1) Low flow/closed circuit
    b. Alveolar concentrations
        (1) All techniques

agents can aid control of the rates and amounts of anesthetic agent delivery.

DETERMINING PHYSIOLOGIC VARIABLES

Physical Principles

Although these principles have been discussed in Chapter 6, the significance of gas analysis during anesthesia delivery for determining physiologic variables is more apparent once understanding of a few simple physical principles is obtained, and so they bear repeating here. First is the principle of conservation of mass, which states that the rate of mass flowing into a system (patient) normally must equal the rate of mass flowing from the system (patient). If these rates are not equal, then the difference between the two must be accounted for by either accumulation (uptake) or reaction (metabolism). In other words, what goes in must come out or accumulate or react. Therefore, every anesthesia delivery system and technique must provide a means of getting a quantity (mass) of gas (respiratory or anesthetic) into and out of a patient, with a minimal amount of unnecessary accumulation and at a sufficient rate to meet various physiologic requirements.

In the patient circuit, the amounts of gaseous components can be measured by numerous techniques. This result can be expressed in units of partial pressure, concentration, or percent concentration and may be displayed digitally as a peak value (end-tidal), an average value, or an instantaneous value. They also can be depicted graphically via strip chart recorder, light-emitting diode (LED) string, or video screen.

Which value is useful will depend upon the determination and calculation of other parameters. For example, from the peak values (end-tidal) of carbon dioxide and the anesthetics, alveolar partial pressures and thence arterial gas tensions can be estimated.[3] Average values are quite adequate to represent background or continuous levels. However, with the instantaneous values of concentration combined with the instantaneous volumetric flow rate, the rate of mass flow can be calculated.[4] As shown in the Appendix at the end of this chapter, by measuring concentrations or partial pressures of the inhaled and exhaled gases and combining those values with the volumetric flow rates of the inhaled and exhaled gases, the rate of mass flowing into and leaving the patient can be calculated (e.g., the rate of anesthetic induction).

For oxygen and carbon dioxide, the difference between these two values (inhaled mass flow − exhaled mass flow) represents oxygen consumption and carbon dioxide production. From these values, respiratory quotient is easily calculated, because it is the ratio of carbon dioxide production to oxygen consumption; thus this indicator of metabolic/nutritional status may be determined easily (Table 4).

For anesthetic agents, the difference between inhaled and exhaled mass flow rates determines the rate of anesthetic uptake. Once the rates of uptake have been determined, cumulative uptakes, total agent utilized, and other variables are easily determined.

As shown in Figure 1, if a mass balance is determined for the airways at steady state, the amount of any constituent entering the lung (inhaled gas and venous blood) must equal the amount of that same constituent leaving the lung (exhaled gas and arterial blood), or accumulate, or react. This also is true if the same principles are applied to the capillaries of the lung.

For the airways, assuming no reactions occur, the difference between the rate at which mass of a constituent (anesthetic) is brought into the lung during inspiration and the rate at which mass is carried from the lung during exhalation will yield the rate of uptake (accumulation) during induction and the rate of elimination during emergence.

For the capillaries (vascular space), the rate of uptake is equal to the difference between the rate at which mass of the constituent flows into the lung via venous return and the rate at which mass flows from the lung via arterial blood. If the volume flow rate (cardiac output, [CO]) is constant, the rate of uptake is equal to the product of flow

Table 4. Determining Physiologic Variables

1. Using oxygen
   a. Cardiovascular
      (1) Cardiac output (Fick principle)
   b. Pulmonary
      (1) $(A\text{-}a)DO_2$
      (2) Shunt (Q_S/Q_T)
   c. Metabolism
      (1) Respiratory quotient (RQ)
      (2) Oxygen consumption
2. Using carbon dioxide
   a. Cardiovascular
      (1) Cardiac output (Fick principle)
   b. Respiratory
      (1) Dead space (V_D/V_T)
      (2) Estimate acid base status $(P_ACO_2 \cong PaCO_2)$
      (3) Ventilation/perfusion relationships
   c. Metabolism
      (1) CO_2 production
      (2) Respiratory quotient
3. Nitrous oxide, volatile anesthetic agents
   a. Cardiovascular
      (1) Cardiac output (Fick principle)
   b. Pulmonary
      (1) Respiration rate

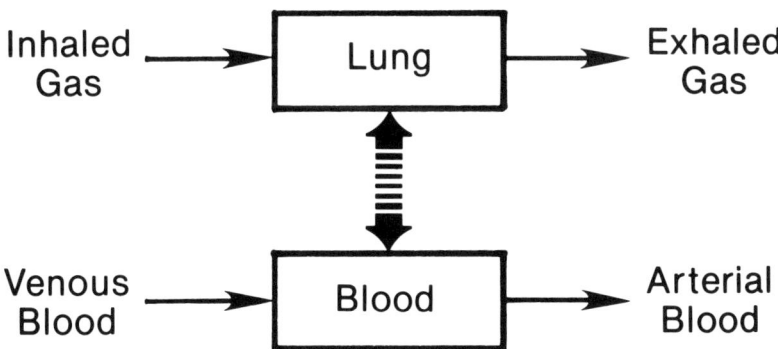

Figure 1. Mass balance in alveolar-capillary interface is shown here schematically.

rate times the difference between the concentration of the constituent in each stream. This is expressed mathematically as the Fick principle for cardiac output (CO = uptake/(Pa-Pv)α). Either the Fick expression or an empirical technique (square root of time model) can be used to estimate cardiac output.

Fick's relationship will enable estimations of cardiac output to be made, if all variables can be measured independently. Analysis of inhaled and exhaled gases in conjunction with end-tidal gas concentrations will enable calculation of rate of uptake and arterial concentration. Unless a mixed venous blood specimen is analyzed, application of this principle is limited and requires that assumptions be made about content of the constituent in the venous blood.

To avoid these limitations, other empirical models must be employed, such as the square root of time model.[5] This model states that the rate of uptake is directly related to the alveolar concentration of the constituent, various partition coefficients, cardiac output, and square root of elapsed time (see Appendix).

In addition to cardiovascular status, parameters relating to respiratory status can be estimated. Ventilation status can be assessed by determination of physiologic dead space (V_D/V_T) using the Bohr equation $V_D/V_T = [(P_{aCO_2} - P_{ECO_2})/P_{aCO_2}]$. Ventilation-perfusion relationships can be assessed using the alveolar gas equation; in addition, alveolar-arterial abnormalities may be determined by knowing alveolar gas concentration.

SUMMARY

With proper measurement of inhaled and exhaled gas concentrations as well as end-tidal concentrations, patient concentrations of oxygen, carbon dioxide, and the volatile anesthetic agents may be inferred; additional information for vigilance monitoring, control of depth of anesthesia, and calculation of physiologic variables can be obtained. From this information, the anesthesiologist will be able to administer improved patient care through more immediate and complete knowledge and control of both equipment and patient function.

REFERENCES

1. GRAVENSTEIN, JS, ET AL: *Section Cutaneous Tissue and Respiratory Gas Measurements: Essential Monitoring in Anaesthesia.* Grune and Stratton, 163–259, 1980.

2. SAIDMAN, LJ AND SMITH, NT: *Monitoring in Anesthesia.* John Wiley & Sons, 1978.
3. NUNN, JF AND HILL, DW: *Respiratory dead space and arterial to end tidal CO_2 tension difference in anesthetized man.* Journal of Applied Physiology 15(3): 383–389, 1960.
4. LAURIA, MJ, ET AL: *A real-time anesthetic data acquisition and processing system. IEEE Trans Biomed Engr* 29:(8)604, 1982 (invited paper).
5. LOWE, HJ AND ERNST, EA: *Uptake and distribution square root model.* In LOWE, HJ AND ERNST, EA: *The Quantitative Practice of Anesthesia.* Williams & Wilkins, Baltimore, 1981.

APPENDIX. MATHEMATICAL FORMULATIONS

The conservation of mass can be expressed mathematically as

(1) $\begin{bmatrix} \text{Rate of} \\ \text{mass flow} \\ \text{(mass/} \\ \text{unit time)} \end{bmatrix} = \begin{bmatrix} \text{Rate of} \\ \text{mass consumed by} \\ \text{reaction} \\ \text{(mass/unit time)} \end{bmatrix} + \begin{bmatrix} \text{Rate of} \\ \text{mass flow} \\ \text{out (mass/} \\ \text{unit time)} \end{bmatrix} + \begin{bmatrix} \text{Rate of} \\ \text{mass accumulation} \\ \text{(mass/unit time)} \end{bmatrix}$

The rate of mass flow (mass/unit time) can be expressed in several ways. For example, it may be the mathematical product of the density ρ (mass/unit volume) times the volumetric flow rate $\dot{V}$ (volume/unit time).

Volumetric flow rate ($\dot{V}$) can be easily measured by a number of techniques (pneumotachograph, respirometer). Density (ρ) is more difficult to determine directly.

Gases at the usual conditions of pressure and temperature of routine anesthesia delivery can be considered to behave ideally and obey the ideal gas law.

The ideal gas law can be simply stated as

(A1) $PV = nRT$

where
- P = partial pressure
- V = volume
- n = number of moles
- R = ideal gas constant
- T = temperature

From this law, concentration (C) can be defined in terms of an ideal gas as the number of moles per unit volume and expressed mathematically as

(A2) $$C = \frac{n}{V} = \frac{P}{RT}$$

Furthermore, density (ρ) is related directly to concentration by molecular weight (M) and can be expressed as

$$(A3) \qquad \rho = CM$$

substituting equation (A2) into equation (A3) yields

$$(A4) \qquad \rho = \frac{MP}{RT}$$

Thus, rate of mass flow can be expressed as

$$(A5) \qquad \omega = \rho\dot{V} = \frac{\dot{V}MP}{RT}$$

In addition to these relationships, Dalton's law of partial pressures relates the partial pressure (P) and percent concentration (%C). This relationship can be expressed in terms of total (atmospheric or circuit) pressure (P_T) as

$$(A6) \qquad \%C = \frac{P}{P_T}(100)$$

From a simple mass balance around the lung capillary (see Figure 1), the rate of mass into lung capillary via venous blood flow and diffusion from the alveolus must equal the rate of mass flow leaving the lung capillary (arterial blood). The mathematic expression for this is Fick's principle of cardiac output.

where
$$(A7) \qquad U = (Pa - Pv) \times \alpha \times CO$$
$$U = \text{rate of uptake}$$
$$Pa, Pv = \text{partial pressures in arterial and mixed venous blood}$$
$$CO = \text{cardiac output}$$
$$\alpha = \text{blood gas solubility coefficient}$$

From a simple volatile agent mass balance as previously described, cardiac output can be estimated using an uptake model such as the square root of time model.

The rate of uptake can be determined from the difference between the rate of mass entering and that of leaving the system (patient);

this is easily accomplished by analysis of concentrations and flow rates of constituents as previously discussed. From the square root of time model, the rate of uptake (U) of an anesthetic agent is a function of the alveolar concentration (C_A), blood gas solubility ($\lambda_{B/G}$), time (τ), and cardiac output (CO) and can be expressed as

$$(A8) \qquad U = C_A \times \lambda_{B/G} \times CO \times \tau^{-1/2}$$

Alveolar concentration (C_A) can be considered to be approximately equal to the end-tidal value (C_{ET}). The blood gas partition coefficient ($\lambda_{B/G}$) is relatively constant for all patients. The only unknown in the equation is cardiac output (CO). However, it is assumed that physiologic shunt, V_D/V_T and distribution space for anesthetic are average values.

Likewise, respiratory variables can be measured in the same manner previously discussed. Respiratory physiologic dead space (V_D/V_T) is easily calculated from the Bohr equation, which can be stated simply as

$$(A9) \qquad V_D/V_T = \frac{PaCO_2 - P_ECO_2}{PaCO_2}$$

where
V_D = physiologic dead space
V_T = total volume
$PaCO_2$ = arterial CO_2 (approximately end-tidal CO_2)
P_ECO_2 = exhaled CO_2 (average mxed value)

Ventilation Perfusion Relationships
Alveolar Gas Equation

$$(A10) \qquad P_{AO_2} = P_{IO_2} - \left[\frac{P_{ACO_2}}{R}\right] + \left[P_{ACO_2} \cdot F_{IO_2} \cdot \frac{(1-R)}{R}\right]$$

where R is the Respiratory Quotient

$$(A11) \qquad R = \frac{\dot{V}_{CO_2}}{\dot{V}_{O_2}}$$

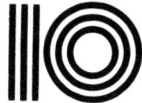

GETTING THE DATA: REDUCING CONFUSION WITH THE COMPUTER

Donald G. Schultz, Ph.D., and
Walter J. Arnell, Ph.D.

The subject of risk in anesthesiology is a topic evident in the literature, and perhaps even more so in the minds of the practitioner. In the ideal case, no complications result from the administration of the anesthetic, and, in fact, it is the responsibility of the anesthesiologist to insure that the ideal case does exist whenever possible. Perhaps the most effective means of preventing a critical incident is development of an early warning system. This chapter deals with a computer-based early warning system that could prove to be the anesthesiologist's greatest ally in everyday as well as crisis situations. The human factors engineering problems concerned with interfaces between such a system and the anesthesiologist are of utmost importance.

If the patient in the operating room is viewed as a complex dynamic system, then early determination of the start of a critical incident may be considered a problem in detection of a system failure. This is a topic under active investigation in areas other than anesthesiology and subject of a 1980 NATO conference on human detection and diagnosis of system failures.[1] The conference was convened to discuss the problems and solutions associated with human ability to cope with failures within complex technical systems.

This was not a medical conference, and no anesthesiologists were in attendance. The types of complex technical systems under discussion included, among others, transportation systems, production processes, nuclear power plants, and communication networks. At issue was the amount of automation necessary or desirable to take advantage of, or to protect against, human intervention in both the normal and crisis modes of operation of these systems. Not at issue in any sense of the word was the question of data processing—quite the contrary. The underlying assumption of the entire conference was that either the human or the automated control system would have available all the data and processed data necessary for the decision-making process.

Unfortunately, the authors are unable to proceed from the conclusions of the NATO conference, simply because data processing is not a significant fact of life in the normal sphere of activity of the anesthesiologist. It is the goal of this chapter to convince the reader that the entire future of anesthesiology is inevitably linked to the use of the digital computer for data processing, information processing, modeling and prediction, and ultimately for control. Human factors problems, more than computer problems, present the most difficult hurdles to be overcome.

This chapter could be devoted entirely to human factors engineering, but as applied to the anesthesiology delivery system with which we are familiar. We feel so strongly that data processing *must* become a part of that delivery system that much of this chapter is devoted to examination of this position. Thus in this chapter, as far as human factors are concerned, we are not dealing with the knobs and dials of the present system. The crucial question is the nature of the interface of the central data display area with the anesthesiologist and the dynamic system of which that individual is a part.

The discussion immediately following this introduction includes the basic assumptions on which this chapter is based and defines a number of terms used throughout, particularly within the context of anesthesiology. Following are discussions on data processing, modeling and prediction, and human engineering. The conclusion is followed by a system test plan that each reader is asked to consider seriously, and even personally.

FOUR BASIC ASSUMPTIONS

Decision Making and Prediction

The first assumption is that the primary function of the anesthesiologist is decision making and prediction and that these two functions are really inseparable. The decisions required usually involve immediate action to cause or to prevent a probable course of action that is expected to occur in the future. Ideally, at least from our point of view, this course of action that is to be affected should be expressible in terms of a change in a measurable variable that is some indication of the inputs to the patient or of the patient status. The key thought here is that making the decision as to the course of action to be taken is a higher level activity than actually carrying out the decision.

Several anesthesiologists assure us that the majority of anesthesiologists agree that decision making is their highest function. Thus, perhaps this assumption need not be mentioned. The assumption is stated here with emphasis because of the well-known comparison with pilots that is so common within the profession. The analogies with which the readers are familiar certainly do hold; but with respect to the primary functions of decision making and prediction, the analogy completely breaks down. The pilot is situated in an environment that has resulted from thousands of man-years of research and development, and the pilot has at disposal sufficient data, processed data, and computational aids so that the plane may fly without the pilot, as on autopilot, or even land with minimal pilot aid, as on an instrument landing. The anesthesiologist is not in this enviable position. The anesthesiologist functions in spite of the operating room environment, instead of being aided by it. It must further be noted that unlike the pilot in the man-engineered system, the anesthesiologist is dealing with a much more complex dynamic physiologic system, totally God-manufactured, the complexities of which are only just beginning to be understood. The variables and parameters of this dynamic system form the diagnostic patterns from which patient status must be evaluated. From a human engineering point of view, the status of instrumentation is primitive, especially if the pilot analogy continues to be the comparison. Note that the only data processing that is routinely done in the operating room is the calculation of heart rate from the electrocardiogram monitor. Clearly the primary function of the anesthesiologist, namely, decision making, must suffer.

Availability of Variables

The second assumption is that, in time, all the variables that the anesthesiologist may wish to have available will actually be available. This is both good news and bad news. In the positive sense, this second assumption is something of an article of faith, based on belief in the combined power of research and the profit motive. It is good to know that in time all the desired data will be there. But the bad news is that there may be too much data to comprehend. Cooper[2] has listed 30 variables that may well prove to be desirable, and time will probably increase the list.

The problem of many variables is particularly difficult when they represent a number of time-dependent events running serially and parallel. A graphic example is the landing of a S/VTOL aircraft on a carrier deck. The pilot must manipulate the aircraft on the x, y, and z axis while coping with wind gusts, tracking a radio beam, maintaining voice communication with air traffic control, and observing a moving carrier deck. Successful landings are possible because the display presentation to the pilot is optimal with respect to the pilot's human processing capabilities.

In the case of the anesthesiologist, the task of maintaining a patient in an ideal status is an analogous activity, in which the goal is the avoidance of a critical event. The information problem is also similar, namely, the presentation of data in a manner to coincide with the anesthesiologist's human data-processing capabilities.

Centralized Displays

The third assumption is that a centralized display will be a marked advantage to the decision maker. The lack of optimal work load versus task performance at the interface between the anesthesiologist and the operating room environment is blatantly obvious. The anesthesiologist is still 100 percent committed to the "scan-interpret-decision" method of operation.[3] Yet concepts of integrated instrument and display design reduce operator-task complexity and are being embraced in a wide variety of system contexts in other fields.

In defense of the anesthesiologist, it must be said that the anesthesiologist is in a sense a victim of those who manufacture equipment. As each new development in the field of anesthesia has occurred, pieces of equipment have been added to the work area in an ad hoc manner to the point that now a typical operation may appear to the uninitiated as considerable disorganization. In fact, it seems so to the anesthesiologist also, and it is perceived as a hindrance to the primary function of decision making.

Computer as Funnel

The last assumption is that a computer will serve as a funnel which will channel all the measured data to a central display area. Furthermore, it is assumed that the addition of a computer will not affect the normal presentation of the measured quantities on whatever type of output device that is normally used to display that quantity. This is not a demanding assumption in terms of hardware. In terms of an operating procedure, this is a fail-safe mechanism that would leave anesthesiologists in their present situation. That is, in case of a computer failure, the anesthesiologist would simply gather the data from the variety of output devices that are now normally used. The type of centralized data, processed data, or processed information display that might ultimately be used is the subject of the next discussion.

The key idea that runs through all the above assumptions is the thought that data are the sacred cow. *Data* are assumed to be the direct output of a transducer or measuring device. Usually these data are in analog form, and before they can be handled by a computer, the data must be passed through an analog to digital converter. This device may or may not be a part of the computer itself. *Processed data* are data that have been put in digital form and processed by the computer. All data and processed data refer to the operation being performed. The words *information* and *information processing* are used here to refer to data that pertain to other cases. For example, if the present operation has been done in the past, you may wish to know if the variations that are apparent in one or more variables are typical of variations that occurred in other successful operations, or if they are an early warning of a crisis situation developing.

There are other properties of the computer that may be of particular importance to the anesthesiologist. The computer never gets bored, nor does its attention wane, nor does it need coffee during the middle of the operation. Its memory is prodigious, as are its recording capabilities. This is in addition to its computational speed and willingness to serve in *exactly* the manner in which the anesthesiologist desires, depending on the software it has been given. Furthermore, as has been stated in this last assumption, if you don't like the computer, just unplug it and proceed in the usual manner.

DATA PROCESSING

The assumption of the use of a computer as a common data output for all machine and patient-monitoring duties is the key idea here. The decision-making arena in which anesthesiologists now find themselves is simply a cluttered mess of equipment and a variety of display mechanisms. Centralization of information would certainly be helpful to the decision-making process. But much more important is the fact that once in digital form, the data can be manipulated in a wide variety of ways.

Before examining the range of possibilities that exist in terms of data processing, let us return briefly to the pilot analogy. Auto pilots have existed for many years, as have the capabilities for instrument landings. Yet there is no thought of flying without a pilot. The reason is that in a decision-making activity, a person acts much like a computer, but a person is much more flexible. Inputs are not through analog to digital converters but through the senses, and as opposed to the computer, the person can manipulate the objects rather than just numbers. The amazing speed and success of the US space program that culminated in the placement of a man on the moon was due in part to an early policy decision to put a man in the space vehicle, even at the rather considerable cost of a life-support system. The message here is not to fear the computer. You will not be replaced or become redundant; but, rather, you will have a fast and attentive slave to serve you, one particularly competent in the area of data processing. To put this portion of the discussion in less general terms, consider the processing that might be done on just one set of data. To be consistent with the other chapters in this book, one might expect that here a machine variable might be used as an example. In a system sense, machine variables are inputs to the patient. Inputs need to be displayed, but it is the effects of the inputs, the patient variables, that might benefit the most from processing. Hence, the signal considered is that received from the electrocardiogram (ECG) monitor. This particular signal is chosen because it is commonly monitored during anesthesia, during surgery, and in recovery and intensive care units. A typical ECG signal is pictured in Figure 1. This signal is usually displayed

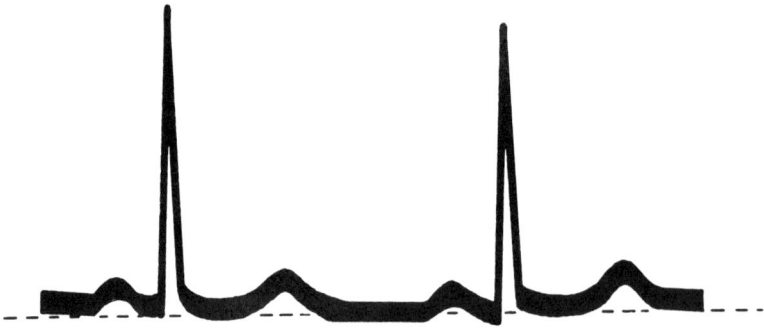

Figure 1. A typical ECG plot for a single cardiac cycle.

on an oscilloscope for each heartbeat of the patient. Additional outputs are a calculated heart rate and an audible signal if the peak amplitude of the ECG exceeds a specified threshold level. Strip chart recordings can also be made if desired.

Gravenstein and coworkers[4] devote an entire section of their book to the subject of electrocardiography in the operating room. The treatment is from a research point of view and is presented in depth. Here, for the purposes of exposition, a simple "for instance" will be given to illustrate the potential power of both data processing and information processing.

The goal of this example is to display changes in the ECG as the patient is stressed by anesthesia and surgery. Thus the first requirement is the establishment of a reference from which changes can be measured. When the patient is brought to the operating room and the ECG monitor is in place, but before anesthesia, a number of heartbeats—say 100—could be recorded and averaged so that the reference ECG can be established within the computer or visually on the oscilloscope. During anesthesia, each ECG pattern could be recorded, and the maximum amplitude for indexing made to coincide with that of the reference waveform. The comparison could be digital, with a resulting numeric measure of the difference between the two waveforms, or both the reference and its comparison could be displayed on an oscilloscope. Dual beam scopes are almost always equipped with a means of displaying the difference between signals applied to their terminals, so that a time-based picture of the difference between the two signals would result. This difference signal, of course, gives a beat by beat measure of the effect of anesthesia on the ECG. If desired, before surgery a second reference could be established, so that at any time during surgery the ECG could be compared with either of the two established references. This error signal could be stored so that additional comparisons could be made. In addition, algorithms now exist that make detection and classification of arrhythmias possible as well.

The reader must realize that once the data processing has been done, a major problem that remains is presentation of the resulting information in a manner useful in the decision-making process; again we are back to the human engineering problem.

Consider now the subject of information rather than data processing. In this example, information processing requires additional stored data within the computer from other similar operations. This may enable the anesthesiologist to rapidly categorize the patient and note what actions in the past have proved to be for the better or for the worse. With this type of information in hand, now is the time for a decision from the anesthesiologist regarding action to be taken.

PREDICTION AND MODELING

The reader may have noted that in the text the word prediction was never mentioned, though it was certainly implied that if error keeps getting worse, serious problems could result. Earlier it was postulated that the patient in the operating room should be viewed as a complex dynamic system. In this discussion, an attempt is made to show that the type of predictions made by anesthesiologists essentially ignore the complex dynamic nature of the human system. The basis of the argument is that no attempt is made to identify the variables of the patient so that these may be taken into account in the prediction process.

A dynamic system is defined as one in which the variables are a function of time. If the variables are not a function of time, the system is said to be static. Clearly, those quantities that determine the status of the patient are quantities or variables that change with time. In order to illustrate the difficulties that are inherent in the prediction of the future value of a variable in a dynamic system, consider the three data points shown in Figure 2. These values have been measured at equally spaced time intervals t1, t2, and t3, and you are asked to predict the value of the variable at time t4. (Here t4 is also equally spaced.)

As indicated in the figure, points P1, P2, and P3 are all in a straight line, and it may seem natural to assume that at t4 the point P4 will also lie on that same line. The actual continuous time trajectory of the variable is shown in Figure 3, and the predicted value of P4 is far from the actual value. And this is a simple dynamic system!

The type of prediction that led to the incorrect value of P4 is much more a curve-fitting technique or a data extrapolation than it is a prediction. In order to be able to predict in a dynamic system, one must know the initial conditions and the values of the parameters that define the system. Consideration of the system from which the trajectory of Figure 3 resulted serves to illustrate the point. The example must be considered in some detail in order to be understood.

The example pictured in Figure 4 is a classical example in mechanics. In that figure, M represents a mass, K a spring, and D a damping element, much like the shock absorber in your car. In this example,

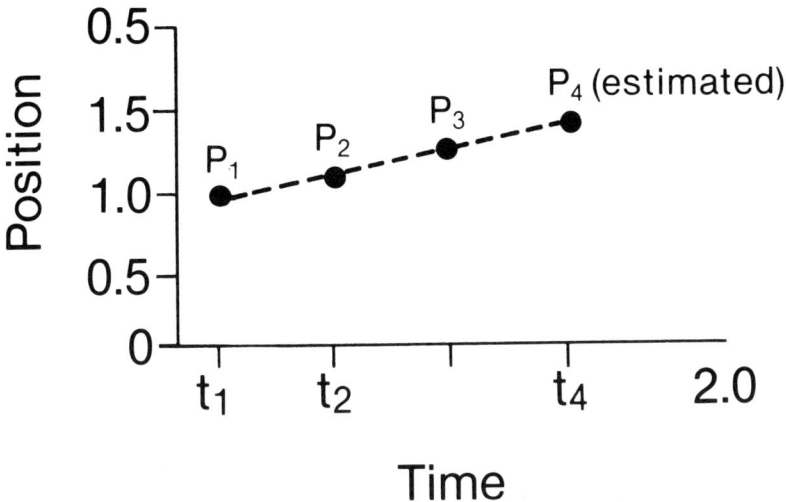

Figure 2. Three recorded data points measured at equally spaced time intervals.

M, K, and D are all assumed to have specific numeric values corresponding to the actual component values in the mechanical system being modeled. Note that in the figure, the initial value of the position variable x is shown to be 0 (zero), and because displacements are of interest, the positive values of x are indicated as being down. The direction of positive force is also downward.

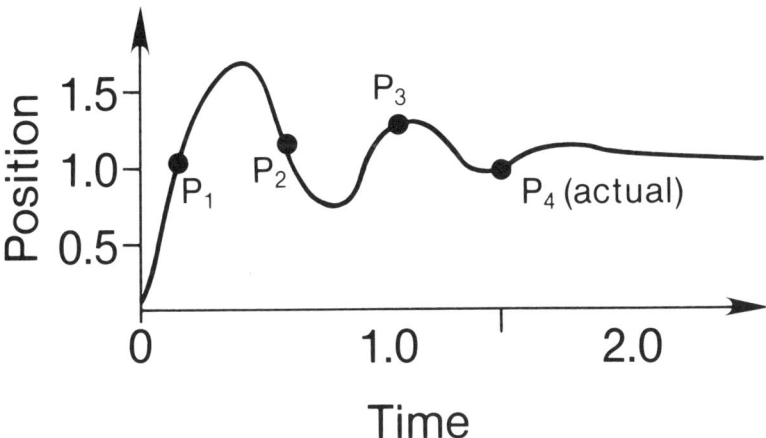

Figure 3. The actual curve from which the data of Figure 3 were taken.

GETTING THE DATA: REDUCING CONFUSION WITH THE COMPUTER   157

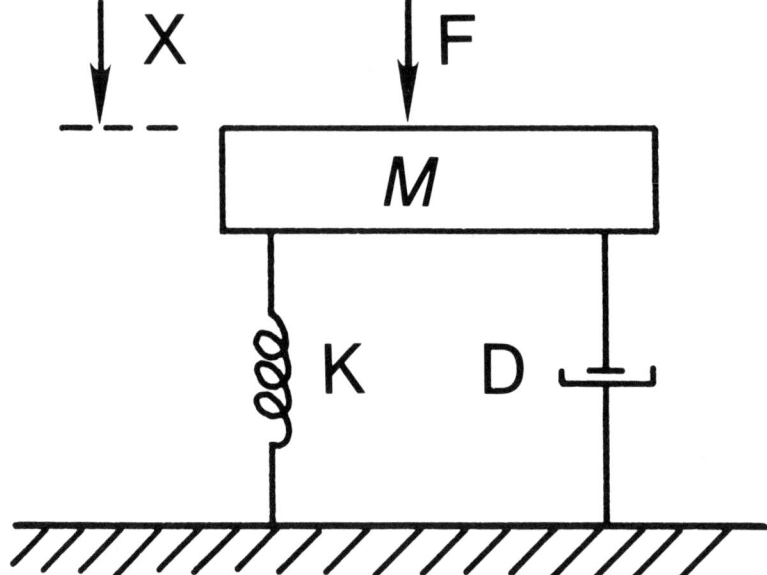

Figure 4. The mechanical system for which the position is plotted in Figure 3 after a constant applied force at time = 0.

If a force F is applied to the mass at time 0, the mass will move, and a plot of x versus time, or x(t) is exactly the trajectory of Figure 3. In this example, the values of M, K, and D have been chosen so that the time response of the position variable is oscillatory.

Ignore the details of the above example if you wish, but note the following facts:

1. Our simple example has a definite structure. The elements that make up the system are connected in a specific way that is detailed in the figure.

2. The mechanical elements are assumed to be *lumped parameters*. An actual spring, for instance, does have mass and not only a spring constant.

3. An *initial condition* was specified. It was the rest or steady state position of the system before the forcing function was applied.

4. A knowledge of x at any one time t is not enough to describe the condition or state of that system at that time. In this example, one also needs to know the velocity. The reason for the incorrect guess on point 4 is that you were not aware that the velocity was changing direction.

5. This system had *one input,* F, *one output,* x(t), and is completely described by two state variables, position and velocity.

6. Sampled values of the position variable could result in an *error* in estimating future values, as with P4.

Statements 1 to 5 above emphasize that the example is indeed a simple one, and statement 6 says that even in simple cases, sampling can be dangerous. Compared with this example, the human physiologic system is orders of magnitude more complicated. There are many inputs and many outputs, with couplings between subsystems that are distributed, rather than lumped parameter systems. Structure is not known in terms of the conventional block diagrams, and system parameters are not specified in terms of numeric constants that may readily become part of a mathematical model. With coupling coefficients undefined, parameters unspecified, and even the system structure uncertain, there is no way that prediction can be done in the normal, analytic sense of the word. It is expected that the availability of an on-line digital computer may eventually aid the decision maker, you, in coping with the prediction problem in the extremely complicated dynamic system represented by the human physiologic system.

HUMAN ENGINEERING

Arguments have been made above concerning the vital need for data processing, information processing, and modeling and prediction. The assumption in each case has been that a computer is available and that the computer will serve as the communication link between the system and the human operator.[5] As noted above, the most formidable problems do not lie with the computer but with developing the interface with the anesthesiologist. This is the human engineering problem, and it is impossible to overstress its importance. The immediate difficulty is that we and the anesthesiologists with whom we have spoken are not completely sure of what data they are presently using in their decision-making process. Thus the problem is not solely a problem to be solved by the human engineer but is necessarily a problem that requires the involvement of both the engineer and the anesthesiologist.

But the problem is compounded by the evolutionary nature of the computer usage postulated above. Once the solution to the data presentation has been accomplished to the mutual satisfaction of both parties, the problem will change, because now processed data must also be accommodated, and then processed information, and modeling and prediction will demand attention.

Before this interaction between engineers and anesthesiologists takes place, all that can be done here is to consider possible alternatives that are suggested by other complex dynamic systems involving a human operator. Design characteristics of consoles that are already in operational use in other complex systems include the following:

1. Many consoles have a reduction in the number of displays, i.e., they combine several variables into a single display. Concepts of display integration coupled with automatic data processing and format techniques improve the human operator's capability to approve, to accept, or to reject an ongoing automatic or semiautomatic functioning system. These integrated display systems are designed with the human operator viewed as a sequential processor with limited capacity.

The example previously used of the S/VTOL aircraft serves to illustrate the point. The human engineered man–machine interface must be such that the display parameters representing the x, y, and z axis, along with wind gusts, radio beam, and so forth must have some modicum of integration for the pilot to cope with the necessary event of getting the aircraft back to earth, or at least to a carrier deck. If pilots had to check each parameter in the "scan-interpret-decision" mode, they wouldn't quite do it right!

Along with the concept of integration, it may be appropriate to use figures of probability of normality instead of the state variables themselves. The presentation of this type of data may be either numerical and/or in the form of geometric figures, as is done in high-performance aircraft and space craft instrumentation.

2. Modeling and predictor display techniques could be employed where necessary. Essentially, such a display provides advanced knowledge of the required controls necessary to maintain the system in an ideal state. The model computes future system status based on what the human operator does with the inputs at the present time. Thus, the ideal control input can be identified. Further, with such a display the anesthesiologist can determine periods when some of the variables will be in a normal state leading to a reduction of observations, and hence work load.

3. Data acquisition time for the operator in the system must be reduced by appropriate display design. A constant design compromise is necessary for the operator to "read" an individual variable at the accuracy required and without mental overload. One must constantly acquire time to "read" other variables in their various forms.

4. During the monitoring process, the computer system should make its own record of the time and variables inspected. If the anesthesiologist is lax in the inspection of a particular state variable, then the software should be designed to prompt for inspection, or the variable may be displayed at preprogrammed times. Implied here is the possible availability of a permanent record.

5. Evidence suggests that during diagnosis in a complex system the phenomenon of "cognitive tunnel vision" occurs.[6] In this situation the operator is inclined to think within a framework of a particular subset of state variables. To circumvent this phenomenon, the computer system must interrogate the anesthesiologist during the diagnostic process, basing its questions on the scanning pattern. Such programmed system behavior is not easy to define or to accomplish.

In summary, the human engineer is concerned with the way in which an operator, here specifically the anesthesiologist, processes information to establish a specified course of action. A relatively "intelligent" integrated display system is proposed to replace the current practice of reading individual ad hoc components.

The next stage beyond the video screen may be a heads up display in which the anesthesiologist is seated facing the patient, and data is presented on a see-through screen to one side of his visual field so that he can maintain tactile contact with the patient. A wide variety of alternatives are possible, and, as noted above, this will be an evolutionary process as more data and processed data become available.

CONCLUSION

This chapter has discussed data presentation, data processing, information processing, and prediction as they refer to a computer-based anesthesiologist support system. The very nature of the topics discussed dictated the use of a digital computer, and such use was one of the initial assumptions stated at the outset. The conclusion, however, is more than just the assumption that a computer will be used as an aid in data presentation and decision making. The conclusion is that the future of anesthesiology is inevitably linked to the use of digital computers. Why? Because the anesthesiologist *is* like a pilot and needs every bit of help available.

Consider the obvious alternative of no computer. As new anesthesia machines are developed and new variables are able to be monitored continuously, the work load of the anesthesiologist can only increase. And even if each new development attempts to reduce the demand on the anesthesiologist, the human factors problems of utilization of continuously increasing amounts of information become insurmountable. Even if no real data processing is done, a computer allows for the presentation of vast amounts of data in a manner that the anesthesiologist demands. The variety of presentation schemes is unlimited, because the choice is simply a question of software.

The critical reader may have observed that the more general question of anesthesia management has not been addressed in this paper, and thus the more general system problem is completely ignored. Perhaps "ignored" is too strong a word. Regardless of what is done in terms of hardware modification and placement, the need for data handling and presentation will always remain.

The Test

A necessary component of any general system design is the specification of a test procedure by which one may judge whether the new system is functioning satisfactorily. Wymore[7] stresses that the test procedure should be chosen before the system is built (no hindsight allowed). Though no formal system design has been proposed here, it is still possible to choose a test procedure that is readily understandable. The test is this: Ten years from now as anesthesiologists schedule their own surgery for their own ailments, will they select a hospital and an anesthesiologist that are able to provide the type of computer support described in this paper? The answer must be yes, if the job has been done right. The problem for all of us is to see that the job is done right.

REFERENCES

1. RASMUSSEN, J AND ROUSE, WB: *Human Detection and Diagnosis of System Failures.* Plenum Press, New York, 1980.
2. COOPER, JB: *Anesthesia management systems.* In GRAVENSTEIN, JS, ET AL (EDS): *Monitoring Surgical Patients in the Operating Room.* Charles C. Thomas, Springfield, IL, 1979.
3. PARKS, DL: *Current workload and emerging challenges.* In Moray, N (ED): *Mental Workload—Its Theory and Measurement.* Plenum Press, New York, 1979.
4. GRAVENSTEIN, JS, ET AL (EDS): *Essential Noninvasive Monitoring in Anesthesia.* Grune & Stratton, New York, 1980.
5. HUCHINGSON, RD: *New Horizons for Human Factors in Design.* McGraw Hill, New York, 1981.

6. MORAY, N: *The role of attention in the detection of errors and the diagnosis of failures of man machine systems.* In RASMUSSEN, J AND ROUSE, WB (EDS): *Human Detection and Diagnosis of System Failures.* Plenum Press, New York, 1980.
7. WYMORE, AW: *Systems Engineering Methodology for Interdisciplinary Teams.* John Wiley & Sons, New York, 1976.

ANESTHESIA VENTILATORS: SPECIAL REQUIREMENTS
Charles W. Otto, M.D.

Controlled mechanical ventilation has become as much a part of modern anesthesia practice as halogenated volatile anesthetics. Yet the changes which have occurred in the operating room ventilator over the years are little appreciated or understood. The energy for delivery of gas to the patient is still primarily obtained from a high-pressure gas source. However, new control devices have allowed increasing sophistication and reliability in mechanical ventilation. In this chapter, many of the capabilities and limitations of current operating room ventilators and what may be coming in the future, including the new technique of high-frequency ventilation, will be discussed.

IDEAL OPERATING ROOM VENTILATOR

The characteristics of an ideal operating room ventilator are listed in general terms in Table 1.

Reliability

Reliable mechanical operation is an obvious first requirement for a medical device that will be expected to support a major life-sustaining bodily function. In addition, a mechanical ventilator must be able to

Table 1. Characteristics of Ideal Operating Room Ventilator

Essential Characteristics
  Reliability
  Versatility
  Compactness
  Ease of Use
  Safety
Desirable Characteristics
  Energy Efficiency
  Monitors
  Feedback Control

provide the desired ventilation regardless of changes in the patient's airway resistance or lung-thorax compliance. This requirement has essentially eliminated pressure-cycled ventilators from the operating room. All the ventilators now in use are either volume cycled or time cycled. Volume- or time-cycled ventilators that are also flow generators are essentially uninfluenced by the patient. However, volume- or time-cycled constant-pressure generators may be influenced by high airway resistance or low lung-thorax compliance. For this reason, many of the older operating room ventilators were unable to provide adequate ventilation for patients requiring high airway pressures.

The ideal operating room ventilator, then, should be a volume- or time-cycled flow generator that can provide reliable tidal volumes unaffected by the patient. It must be recognized that the tradeoff for this reliability is that such ventilators have no means of compensating for leaks. Patient ventilation will decrease if a leak develops in the system. Consequently, extreme vigilance on the part of the anesthesiologist is necessary to guard against such an occurrence (see discussion on safety).

Versatility

Ideally, an operating room ventilator should be able to be used for a neonate or a 200 kg adult. However, small children and neonates require small tidal volumes at high frequencies with low inspiratory flows. Many ventilators designed for adults (including most of the current generation of operating room ventilators) either cannot or only poorly meet these requirements. Ventilators now exist for use in intensive care units (ICUs) that are able to provide adequate ventilation for these extremes of body size. Future operating room ventilators should incorporate systems capable of ventilating the very small infant as well as the adult.

Most of the improvements in ventilator technology in the past few years have occurred in machines designed for use in the ICU. These ventilators are designed as nonrebreathing, open-circuit systems. Much of this technology could be immediately adaptable to the operating room if there were general agreement to use open-circuit systems. However, semiclosed and closed-circuit anesthesia retain popularity among a significant number of anesthesiologists. Therefore, any ventilator for use in the operating room must be compatible with these techniques. This has usually meant that operating room ventilators are designed as a bellows in a box where the interior of the bellows is connected to the anesthesia circuit and the bellows is compressed by a separate high-pressure gas source. Some variation on the bellows in a box is likely to be retained in future operating room ventilators, but driving and control mechanisms will become more sophisticated.

Most ICU ventilators now provide the user with a choice of ventilatory modes, including a few or all of the following: controlled, assisted, intermittent mandatory (IMV), mandatory minute volume (MMV), or spontaneous ventilation. In the operating room, most of these modes are superfluous. Unless current anesthetic techniques change greatly in the future, there seems little reason to include more than controlled respiration and the ability for spontaneous respiration in the ventilator-anesthesia circuit. However, positive end expiratory pressure (PEEP) is a ventilatory modality which is now firmly established in respiratory care both in and out of the operating room. It is to be expected that all future operating room ventilators will have systems to provide PEEP when it is indicated.

Compactness

With the increase in monitors and other equipment in the modern operating room, compactness of the mechanical ventilator is not only desirable but essential. Fortunately, the development of fluidic control devices for gases and microchips for electronic controls has already significantly reduced the size of ventilators. This is a trend that is likely to continue in the future, enabling integration of the ventilator into the anesthesia machine or increasing its portability.

Ease of Use

The perfect piece of equipment to do the job at hand is useless if it cannot be operated. As we require more sophisticated operating room ventilators to enable us to manage patients with more severe illnesses, the machines will inevitably become more complex. This will require a greater effort on the part of the anesthesiologist to understand the equipment being used. However, it will also require a significant effort on the part of manufacturers to make the equipment user friendly (to borrow a term from computer technology). Modular components and circuit boards will make servicing easier, but increased complexity will require improved service networks to provide advice and expertise. Although the possibility of transmission of respiratory pathogens from ventilator components is remote under usual operating room conditions, it is important that parts which are in contact with patient gases be easily disassembled for cleaning and/or sterilization.

In order to maintain ease of use with increasing complexity, it is likely that computer technology will be used. Descriptions of ventilator function will be stored in an attached microcomputer and will be displayed on a screen. Instructions for ventilator settings will be typed on a keyboard and automatically carried out. During ventilation, the screen will display internal and external monitoring information and lead the user through troubleshooting should problems develop.

Safety

Automatic monitors and alarms cannot (and should not be expected to) replace the anesthesiologist's clinical monitoring of the patient. However, even an anesthesiologist's vigilance can be distracted, and automatic backup systems are highly desirable. Assuming the ventilator is a volume- or time-cycled flow generator which is uninfluenced by patient lung characteristics, it is imperative that leaks in the system be detected. Most commonly, this is accomplished by monitoring the pressure generated in the patient circuit and sounding an alarm if a preset pressure is not reached. This is an effective system for major leaks or total disconnections but can miss smaller leaks. Some current ventilators have an additional visual alarm. If the bellows is filled from below (against gravity) during the expiratory cycle, leaks of gas from the circuit in excess of fresh gas inflow will not return the bellows to its fully extended position. Consequently, the bellows will eventually collapse (slowly or quickly, depending on the size of the leak). The falling bellows provides an additional visual alarm to a leak in the system.

A better (but technically more difficult) alarm is to measure the tidal or minute volume. The most reliable system would measure volume between the ventilator circuit and the patient. Next best would be to compare the volumes exiting in the circuit to those entering. Even monitoring volumes exiting the circuit alone provides more information than only pressure monitoring. The author believes that because hypoventilation and/or inadvertent disconnections can have such disastrous consequences, all ventilator systems should be monitored at least for circuit pressure and preferably for both pressure and volume.

Another concern when using ventilators that are not influenced by the patient's lung characteristics is the possibility of developing extremely high airway pressures. Most ICU ventilators are equipped with a pressure-limiting system attached to an alarm. When the pressure limit is reached, an alarm sounds and the remainder of the tidal volume is exhausted to the room or the ventilator immediately cycles into an expiratory mode. Because sudden development of high airway pressures is not likely under the controlled conditions of anesthesia, most operating room ventilators do not have this safety feature. Most anesthesia systems are equipped with pressure gauges to monitor developed system pressure. It would seem highly desirable to incorporate this pressure monitoring into an alarm system that would warn of increasing pressures necessary for ventilation. This would serve as a guide to the anesthesiologist to look for potential complications, such as pneumothorax, accumulating secretions, or kinked endotracheal tubes.

Energy Efficiency

In this age of inflation and rising medical costs, it is desirable that all equipment be kept as efficient as possible. This is a major argument for the use of closed-circuit anesthesia. Similarly, consideration should be given in the future to conservation of the energy necessary for driving the ventilator. In most of the commonly used operating room ventilators in the United States, a volume of gas (usually oxygen) equal to the minute ventilation is wasted in the process of compressing the bellows. It would seem that a more efficient system of compressing the bellows could be devised.

Monitors

Future anesthesia systems will likely incorporate additional monitoring devices for respiratory function. Oxygen and carbon dioxide monitoring have been discussed in detail in other chapters. Inspired or expired oxygen concentration monitoring is now common practice and will continue to be used. New uses for monitoring end-tidal carbon dioxide are being described, and carbon dioxide monitors may become an integral part of the anesthesia-ventilator system. In addition, the pressure and volume measurements will be used to calculate and to display airway resistance and lung-thorax compliance.

Feedback Control

Servo control of ventilator function is already a reality in some ICU ventilators that are able to monitor inspiratory flow rates and volumes during a breath, compare them to the control settings, and then make any necessary adjustments. This technology is sure to be brought into the operating room. Automatic control of arterial carbon dioxide by the ventilator could be easily accomplished by connecting carbon dioxide sensors to the ventilator. Under most circumstances in the operating room, end-tidal carbon dioxide could be used as a close approximation of the arterial carbon dioxide. However, it is well recognized that in severe respiratory disease, end-tidal carbon dioxide may not be a good reflection of arterial carbon dioxide. Consequently, it is likely that widespread use of automatic carbon dioxide control will await the development of accurate in vivo carbon dioxide sensors.

VENTILATOR AND THE ANESTHESIA MACHINE

Ventilator as an Accessory

In the United States, the operating room ventilator has developed as an accessory to the anesthesia machine. In some cases, it has been permanently attached to the machine by the user, but the devices were designed so that they could be moved from machine to machine. This portability provides the advantages of not requiring a ventilator for every anesthetizing location and ease of replacement should the device need servicing. However, the ventilator as a separate unit increases the chances that users may find themselves in a situation in which they are not familiar with the device to be used. In addition, as an accessory, the ventilator tends to be removed (to a lesser or greater extent) from the anesthesiologist's scanning and visual range. This increases the potential for critical incidents that could lead to complications.

Recently, anesthesia machines have become available in which ventilator controls are integrated into the basic machine unit. In these systems, the controls and alarms are close to other machine controls and the bellows are mounted in a visually prominent place. These systems provide an important advantage in allowing more consistent interaction with the device by the user and should decrease the frequency of critical incidents. The loss of portability in this arrangement is not a major problem inasmuch as modern anesthetic techniques generally dictate that mechanical ventilation capabilities be available at nearly all anesthetizing locations. However, integration of the ventilator into the anesthesia machine emphasizes the importance of versatility in ventilator design. If it remains necessary to substitute special ventilators for small children or patients with low lung-thorax compliance, then system complexity will be greatly increased and may actually increase the frequency of critical incidents.

Ventilator as Anesthesia Machine

Although integration of controls into the anesthesia module is a step forward, the ventilator still basically remains an accessory to the main gas delivery system. Early attempts to completely combine the ventilator and anesthetic gas delivery systems were not met with much enthusiasm. However, many of the early problems have been or could be solved with modern technology. The anesthesia machine of the future may become a modified ventilator.

Accurate high-pressure air-oxygen and nitrous oxide-oxygen blenders make the choice of basic gases easy and reliable. A few present ventilators have low-pressure gas systems which allow the use of standard volatile agent vaporizers. The development of accurate high-flow vaporizers and injector systems for volatile anesthetics will permit more versatility in adding inhalation anesthesia to ventilator systems. Nearly all ICU ventilators in current use provide a mechanism for spontaneous ventilation through the use of reservoirs or demand valves. Consequently, it is now feasible for the ventilator to function as a gas source regardless of the mode of ventilation.

The last major problem to overcome in allowing the ventilator to function as an anesthesia machine is making the system compatible with closed or semiclosed circuits. This would require adding a soda lime canister to the circuit and developing a method of channeling scavenged exhaled gases back to the ventilator. These are not insurmountable problems.

The advantage of the ventilator as an anesthesia machine is that it would completely integrate the gas delivery system regardless of the mode of ventilation, simplifying the equipment now in use. It would also allow more sophisticated ventilation techniques to be used in the operating room. Both of these are desirable goals.

HIGH-FREQUENCY VENTILATION

High-frequency ventilation (HFV) is a new experimental mode of mechanical ventilation which uses frequencies varying from 1 to 40 Hz (60 to 2400 breaths per minute) and tidal volumes equal to or less than anatomic dead space. The mechanisms by which HFV can provide adequate gas exchange have not been proven but probably involve some type of enhanced molecular diffusion within the tracheobronchial tree. Because the mechanisms are unclear, numerous mechanical systems have been developed for HFV. Each is somewhat different from the others.

In an attempt to bring some order to the field, most investigators have tacitly agreed on a terminology for the most frequently used systems. This terminology is primarily descriptive of the type of system used for ventilation but also roughly defines the range of frequency at which the system works. High-frequency positive pressure ventilation (HFPPV) was the original HFV and is the least used in the United States. It depends on a high-pressure gas source directing flow into the airway through a pneumatic valve. Frequencies usually range from 60 to 120 breaths per minute. High-frequency jet ventilation (HFJV) has been studied extensively in the United States. A solenoid or fluidic valve directs the driving gas to a small orifice jet placed within the airway. Frequencies range from 100 to 1000 breaths per minute with frequencies of 100 to 400 breaths per minute being most common. In both HFPPV and HFJV, exhalation occurs passively owing to lung recoil at the end of inspiration. High-frequency oscillation (HFO) refers to a system in which gas in the airway is oscillated by means of a reciprocating piston or diaphragm with fresh gas intake and carbon dioxide removal being accomplished by a bias flow through the system. Frequencies range upward from 600 breaths per minute with 900 to 1500 breaths per minute being most commonly used.

Although these systems are all different, they do have some common requirements which are different from conventional ventilators. The most important difference from present ventilators is that the system must have a very small internal compliance. If ventilation is to occur with very small tidal volumes, a significant portion of each breath cannot be lost to the patient by being compressed within the tubing of the machine. Consequently, high-frequency ventilators are not just conventional ventilators run at high rates.

Although it must be emphasized that HFV is still an experimental technique, it does appear that it will come into increasing use in the next few years. The systems most likely to be clinically available will be HFJV systems with the jet located in the lumen of special endotracheal tubes or at the proximal orifice of the endotracheal tubes. Such systems may provide advantages over conventional ventilation in patients with bronchopleural fistulae. It is also possible for these systems to provide adequate ventilation with less cardiovascular depression than conventional ventilation. The largest early application of HFJV may be in the operating room. It can be used very well during bronchoscopy and laryngeal surgery in a manner similar to the Sanders technique. The ability to ventilate through a very small tube provides obvious advantages to the surgeon during operations on the trachea and major bronchi. The lack of brain movement during HFV gives it an advantage during microscopic neurosurgery. Ventilation can be provided through a small catheter placed percutaneously through the cricothyroid membrane and may provide protection against aspiration. This could be very valuable in cases of orofacial trauma.

The major disadvantage of the use of HFJV in the operating room is the inability to use volatile anesthetics. High-pressure blenders will allow the use of nitrous oxide-oxygen mixture as the driving gas, but volatile anesthetics will not be available with these systems in the near future. In addition, these are open-circuit systems and are not compatible with closed-circuit anesthesia. Both these disadvantages could potentially be overcome with HFO systems, but such HFO seems unlikely to be in wide clinical use in the near future.

In summary, HFV is an experimental new ventilation technique that seems likely to enter clinical practice in the next few years. As with any other new technique, it will be some time before its proper place in the medical armamentarium is determined.

SECTION 3

PROTOTYPES FOR THE FUTURE

The ultimate anesthesia delivery system has yet to be invented. Described in this section are the parochial best bets. Today a practicing anesthesiologist must be a true troglodyte to deny that patient safety cannot be improved by the mechanism of applied engineering to the field. Alabama, Arizona, Massachusetts, and Utah are some of the areas where new machine development is being pursued. The Alabama system focuses on safe closed-circuit anesthesia delivery as an important factor in new system design. The Arizona group is a multidisciplinary group, redesigning the entire anesthesia delivery system with modularity and human factors as prime considerations. Concerns about reliability, simplicity, and the ability of the anesthetist to override automatic functions are salient factors of emphasis. The Massachusetts General group has long been a leader in the field. The Boston Anesthesia System, one of the first attempts to incorporate truly new and innovative thinking in the area in decades, is a result of a design that was centered around the microprocessor. The functions and operation of the system are based upon the results of studies defining causes of human error in the operating room. Control of the anesthetic through the Utah system, with its emphasis on computer control, is more directly related, via the technology of feedback control, to the patient's status than to the machine.

What will be the eventual outcome? Most likely it will be an integration of these various ideas into a unit acceptable to the physician and with markedly improved safety for the patient.

Burnell R. Brown, Jr.

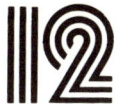

THE ALABAMA AUTOMATED CLOSED-CIRCUIT ANESTHESIA PROJECT

Jeffry A. Spain, M.D.,
Thomas C. Jannett, M.S., and
Edward A. Ernst, M.D.

The Alabama Automated Closed-Circuit Anesthesia Project, which began in late 1980, has as its goal the development of computer-based automatic control technology for the administration of closed-circuit anesthesia. As outlined in Chapter 1 of this volume, the closed-circuit technique permits—in fact, necessitates—precise measurements of several physiologic processes and the quantitative administration of oxygen and anesthetic agents based on these measurements.

To briefly review, consider a case in which an oxygen–volatile agent anesthetic is being administered using closed-circuit anesthesia. In addition to the usual tasks of clinical anesthesia, the anesthesiologist needs to monitor and to control three processes: 1) oxygen delivery, 2) volatile agent delivery, and 3) ventilation.

OXYGEN DELIVERY

The rate of oxygen delivery is determined by the rate of oxygen consumption by the patient. The anesthesiologist measures the end-expiratory anesthetic circuit volume and oxygen concentration and adjusts the oxygen flow to maintain a constant circuit volume. In this situation, because the circuit is closed, the rate of oxygen delivery must equal the rate of oxygen consumption by the patient. The anesthesiologist may compare the oxygen consumption measurement to a theoretical model which states that the oxygen consumption should equal 10 × (patient mass in kg)$^{3/4}$ ml per minute at 37° C.[1] If the measured and predicted oxygen consumptions differ significantly, the anesthesiologist knows that some problem exists. If the measured oxygen consumption exceeds the predicted amount, the anesthesiologist may consider causes such as circuit leak, hyperthyroidism, and malignant hyperthermia. In the opposite case, the anesthesiologist would consider hypothermia or circulatory failure.

VOLATILE AGENT DELIVERY

The rate of volatile agent delivery is determined by the rate of volatile agent uptake by the patient. The volatile agent is usually administered by injecting it in liquid form into the exhalation limb of the circuit at a rate required to maintain a constant end-expiratory concentration. Because the circuit is closed, the rate of volatile agent delivery must equal its rate of uptake by the patient, and the measured circuit concentration remains constant. To guide the anesthesiologist in the administration of the volatile agent, the square root of time model[2] of uptake and distribution is useful. This model predicts that the rate of anesthetic uptake is the product of the arterial anesthetic concentration, the cardiac output, and the reciprocal of the square root of the elapsed time. Differences between actual and predicted rates of uptake are generally due to variations in cardiac output from the predicted value and may signify that the depth of anesthesia is inappropriately light or deep or that some problem exists within the cardiovascular system.

VENTILATION

The rate of ventilation is determined by the rate of carbon dioxide production by the patient. The anesthesiologist measures the end-expiratory carbon dioxide concentration and adjusts the ventilatory frequency and tidal volume so that this concentration remains constant at a desired level, usually 5 ml per dl (5 percent), or about 40 torr. The theoretic minute ventilation necessary to achieve this concentration depends on the patient's carbon dioxide production and physiologic dead space. Carbon dioxide production depends, in turn, on the product of oxygen consumption and the respiratory quotient. Abnormalities in the respiratory quotient and dead space will cause discrepancies between the actual and predicted end-expiratory carbon dioxide concentrations for a given minute ventilation rate. Carbon dioxide absorber malfunction or depletion would also need to be considered.

USE OF COMPUTER

The feasibility of closed-loop feedback techniques depends upon the measurement accuracy and reliability for the variable to be controlled. Also, it must be possible to make the adjustments required to regulate the variable at the desired level. Inasmuch as the control of oxygen delivery, volatile agent delivery, and ventilation is based on relatively simple measurements and adjustments, it should be possible to control each of these processes automatically in an appropriately instrumented closed-circuit anesthesia system. In each case, a theoretic model is available to use as a basis for the development of the necessary control procedures.

The use of the computer for repetitive measurements, control procedures, and data storage would free the anesthesiologist from these tasks and would provide less erratic control.[3]

SYSTEM DESCRIPTION

The project was divided into three stages: development of the hardware and control algorithms, bench and animal laboratory testing, and clinical trials. As of this writing, hardware development has been completed. An overview of the equipment currently assembled is presented.

The system was constructed mainly of standard anesthesia equipment modified for computer control. As shown in Figure 1, a standard anesthesia gas machine was used. Oxygen, air, and nitrous oxide flowmeters were left in place along with a standard circle absorber system. The volatile agent vaporizers were removed, except for a copper kettle left in place for backup purposes. An Air Shields Ventimeter ventilator was mounted on the circle system. Because this ventilator uses a rising, rather than a hanging, spirometer bellows, it is possible to continuously monitor the anesthetic circuit volume with great sensitivity. In fact, even small changes in intrathoracic volume occurring with the patient's cardiac cycle are reflected as small bellows displacements.

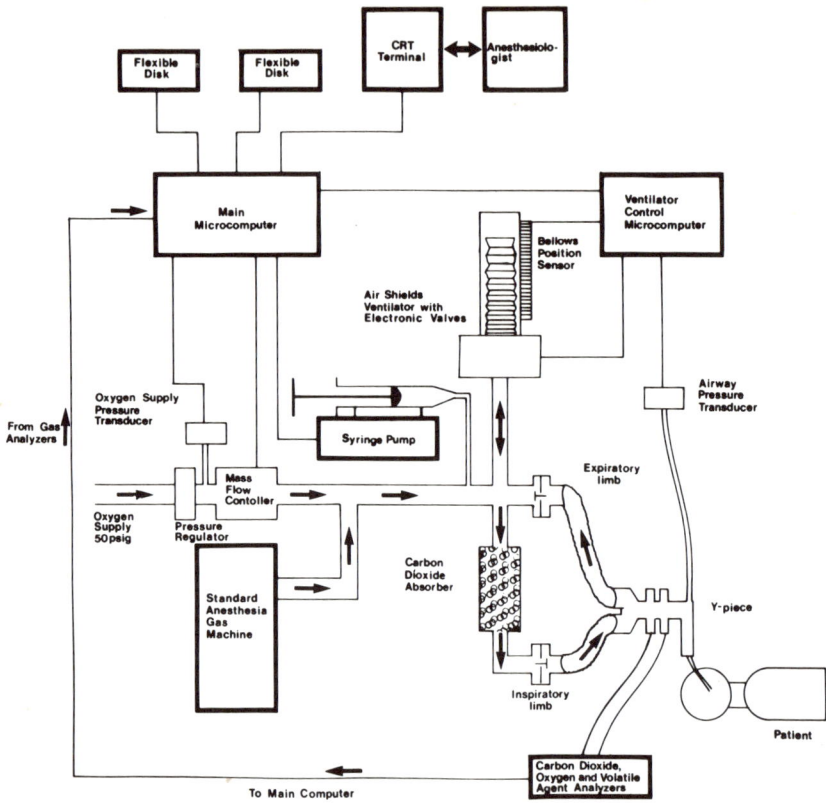

Figure 1. The Alabama Automated Closed-Circuit Anesthesia System.

To facilitate measurement of patient oxygen consumption and to control oxygen delivery, a position sensor was added to the Air Shields bellows canister. The sensor consisted of a stack of 80 light-emitting diode-phototransistor pairs. A small reflective strip of aluminum was then mounted on the top plate of the spirometer bellows so that the phototransistor adjacent to the top of the bellows would be activated at any given time. The position sensor was interfaced to the ventilator control microcomputer, making it possible to read the bellows position and circuit volume to within 17 ml over a 1400 ml range. To allow oxygen flow adjustments, a thermal mass flow controller was added to the gas machine. Its output was piped through a rotameter to allow visual inspection of the oxygen flow and then into the common outlet of the gas machine. The mass flow controller was driven from a 20 psig pressure regulator and was monitored by a pressure transducer to provide a warning of supply gas failure. Both the thermal mass flow controller and the pressure transducer had interfaces with the main microcomputer.

To measure patient anesthetic uptake and to control volatile agent delivery, a volatile agent analyzer was added to the circuit at the Y piece, with an interface to the main computer. Initially an Engstrom EMMA was used, although its sensitivity to water vapor posed a problem. A syringe pump was added to inject volatile agents directly into the expiratory limb of the breathing circuit. The pump's timing circuitry was modified for computer control and was supplied with an interface to the main computer. The use of a syringe pump allows precise regulation of the anesthetic dose and permits visual inspection of the total dose administered.

To evaluate patient ventilation, an infrared carbon dioxide analyzer was added to the circuit at the Y piece, with an interface to the main computer. To allow automatic adjustment of ventilation, the Air Shields ventilator was further modified by replacing its pneumatic timing device with electronic solenoid valves, with an interface to the ventilator control computer. These valves enabled the tidal volume, respiratory frequency, and I:E ratio to be set to values required to regulate the carbon dioxide concentration. A pressure transducer was connected to the circuit at the Y piece and supplied with an interface to the computer for monitoring airway pressure.

Also, the main computer had interfaces with two flexible disk drives for program and data storage, a printer for hard copy output, and a CRT terminal, which permitted interaction with the anesthesiologist. All components were mounted on the anesthesia gas machine, with the exception of the main computer, disks, printer, and CRT, which were placed on an attached cart.

Software to allow control of all the devices with interfaces to the two computers, as well as communication between the computers, is being developed. A simple proportional integral-derivative control algorithm for oxygen delivery has been written and tested in laboratory animals. The controller adjusts the oxygen flow to maintain a predetermined circuit volume. Recordings of oxygen uptake and circuit volume during a dog experiment are shown in Figure 2. Anesthesia was induced and was maintained with pentobarbital sodium. The controller adjusted the oxygen flow to regulate the end-expiratory spiro-

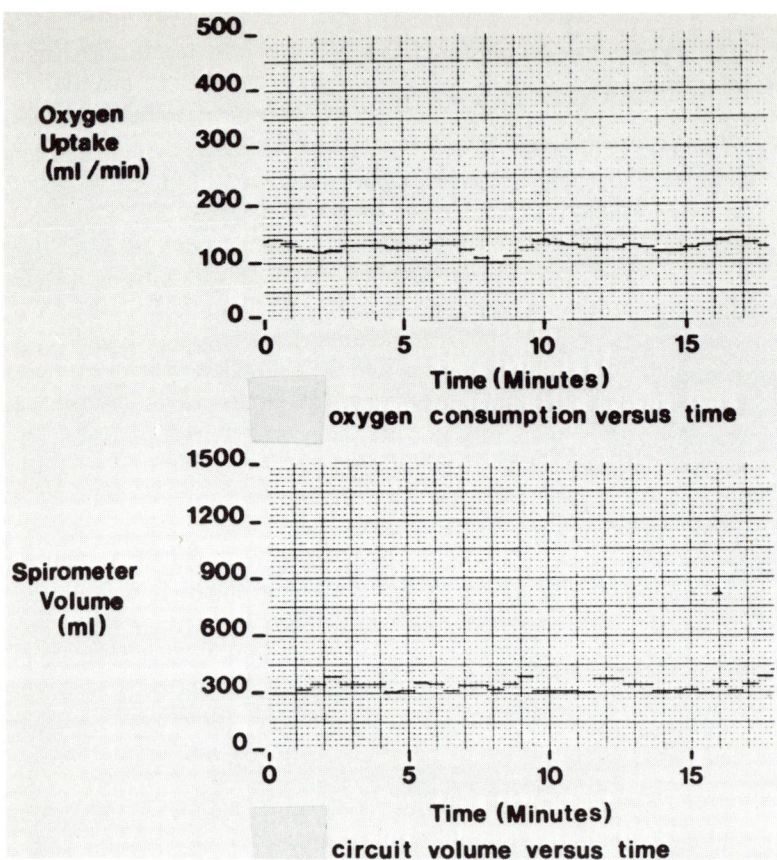

Figure 2. Recordings of measured circuit volume and corresponding automatic oxygen delivery during closed-circuit anesthesia for a 25 kg dog. The predicted oxygen uptake was 112 ml per minute.

meter measurement at the desired value of 1200 ml. Although the accuracy of the oxygen uptake measurements was limited by the resolution of the circuit volume measurements, the experimental measurements were close to the predicted volume of 112 ml per minute (O_2 uptake = 10 $kg^{3/4}$ ml per minute).

COMMENTS

One of the reasons that closed-circuit anesthesia has not gained in popularity is the fact that its administration using manual methods requires more effort than that for high-flow techniques. With high flows one can set the flowmeters and vaporizer and leave them unattended except for infrequent adjustments, but much monitoring data is lost. With a closed circuit, the flowmeter adjustment and the liquid injection process must receive frequent attention to maintain a constant circuit volume and volatile agent concentration. The application of automatic control technology to the administration of closed-circuit anesthesia will greatly diminish the amount of effort needed for its delivery. Furthermore, the measurement and recording of the physiologic data available with the closed-circuit technique will be made more precise, more systematic, and less time-consuming for the anesthesiologist. Thus the automated system will help make closed-circuit anesthesia a more controlled and convenient technique for both the clinician and the researcher.

REFERENCES

1. BRODY, S: *Bioenergetics and Growth.* Reinhold, New York, 1945.
2. LOWE, HJ, ET AL: *Closed system anesthesia.* Anesthesiol Rev 1:11, 1974.
3. SHEPPARD, LC AND KOUCHOUKOS, NT: *Computers as monitors.* Anesthesiology 45(2): 250–259, 1976.

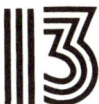

THE ARIZONA PROGRAM: DEVELOPMENT OF A MODULAR, INTERACTIVE ANESTHESIA DELIVERY SYSTEM

Warren R. Jewett, Sc.D.

In 1975, a group of anesthesiologists and engineers at the University of Arizona undertook a program to develop a fully integrated approach to anesthesia delivery. The original concept for an Arizona System centered on design and fabrication of hardware and support instrumentation for creation of a new anesthesia machine. However, it was soon evident that a more important starting place was examination of the extant philosophy and mechanics by which anesthesia is administered. From this study and critique there emerged a new rationale—the present basis for the Arizona System.

Although the processes of anesthesia and the techniques of its delivery are complex, there are four basic phases into which it may be divided:

1. Determination of the parameters by which a particular anesthetic agent is to be delivered and setting initial control variables.
2. Monitoring of depth of anesthesia and alteration of the patient's physiologic functions owing to anesthetics.
3. Intervention with appropriate therapeutic agents to modify the patient's physiological status.

4. Surveillance of the aforementioned processes in order to provide adequate documentation of all events in a comprehensive patient record.

The four phases above have become the targets for research at Arizona. Studies are underway to accomplish those objectives by identifying appropriate methodologies, clearly defining desired component functions, and determining the requisite specifications for the development of the necessary subsystems to be incorporated into an integrated anesthesia delivery system. Once the criteria become clear, "state of the art" technology is examined to determine its applicability to, and compatibility with, system elements. Performance criteria, design concepts, and the hardware itself will determine whether each device is a stand-alone component or is appropriate for integration into a larger system. In all cases, the investigator's primary concerns are to create a design that will insure safety and efficacy with greatest possible utility. There is no desire on the part of the researchers involved to invent or to develop hardware for any part of the system for which there may be an acceptable component already available.

In working toward the goal of an integrated system, four specific areas of research have emerged. The first of these is a systems and human factors study of the interactive relationships among anesthesiologist, patient, and equipment. A second area of investigation is the development and application of appropriate sensor technology, with particular emphasis on patient interfacing.[1] Third, technology is being defined and evaluated for all additional phases of anesthesia delivery. Finally, the fourth division of research deals with automation and feedback control. This entails analysis of computer operations as well as designing for ease of manual override and control.

HUMAN INTERACTION

The folklore regarding operating room procedures, requisite equipment, and the environment in which anesthesiologist-patient-machine interaction takes place is being reexamined. Elements within this triad are being investigated for a more thorough understanding of the complexities of the action/reaction process. It is hoped that the studies will provide techniques and instrument designs that will facilitate these interactions with increased utility and patient safety.

In the operating room, the anesthesiologist is inundated with a constant barrage of information from patient, monitors, anesthesia apparatus, and surrounding environment. How all of this data is processed and the use to which it is put must be thoroughly understood. In order to do this, examination of the decision-making processes confronting anesthesiologists and their assimilation/response techniques is being analyzed.

It has become necessary in such a study to recognize and to separate extraneous data and distraction from that information indispensable for safe, effective patient management. Once this identification has been made, machine, monitors, and sensors can be designed to accommodate anesthesiologists' needs. Much of the decision-making process may ultimately be computer modeled with total automation of some processes.

It is anticipated that guidelines generated by this study will be used for the creation of an anesthesia delivery system that can function with a minimum of effort on the part of the anesthesiologist. Monitored data with preliminary analysis and trend lines can be presented via visual displays and/or audio-annunciators in a format determined to be least confusing to the operator. Required responses should be simple, direct interactions with machine and patient. Finally, sound technology, reliability, and precision in the instrumentation of choice are obvious criteria.

SENSORS

The key to the development of any anesthesia delivery system is the identification and utilization of appropriate sensors. These devices provide the means for monitoring machine performance and reflecting the depth of anesthesia along with detection of physiologic changes within the patient. Emphasis has been placed upon the evaluation and development of gas concentration sensors and flowmeters. Investigations of improved techniques for monitoring patient variables of blood pressure, electroencephalogram, and electrocardiogram are also part of the program.

In evaluating sensors, an attempt has been made to identify those types which combine rugged design with accuracy, reproducibility, and maximum reliability. Those devices not readily correctable for thermal- or pressure-induced drift were eliminated from consideration.

Gas Sensors

Commercially available gas sensors have limitations which restrict their acceptability for inclusion in new anesthesia delivery systems. Among the drawbacks to use of these devices are size, cost, accuracy, response time, stability, and, of particular concern, moisture and temperature sensitivity. Considerable effort has been expended to investigate new technologies and to provide, when necessary, the engineering to incorporate appropriate sensors into the system.

Flueric Oscillator Sensor

One type of gas sensor being developed is a flueric jet edge resonator oscillator.[2] This type of oscillator (Fig. 1 and Fig. 2) consists of a jet edge (wedge) surrounded by a resonating cavity. At a constant flow rate, the gas stream emerges from an inlet nozzle into the oscillator. Approximately 98 percent of this stream continues to flow through the unit and out the exhaust. The remaining 2 percent strikes the sharp edge, producing an edge tone oscillation, which forces the stream into one of the cavities; there the stream attaches to the wall (Coanda effect). This phenomenon creates an increase in momentum and mass flow, which produces a pressure pulse in the cavity.

Because the pressure is now greater in one of the two cavities, the direction of flow switches toward the cavity of lower pressure. The resultant oscillating pressure pulses are measured with a pressure transducer, which is connected to one cavity via a small pressure channel. The oscillations are self-maintained and depend upon the particular geometry of the oscillator, temperature, molecular weights, and ratios of specific heats (C_p/C_v) of the gas. Oscillators are approximately one centimeter square in size and produce a 30 kHz frequency with air.

A gas sensor consists of two such oscillators operating in parallel. A reference gas is drawn through one oscillator, and the unknown gas mixed in the reference gas is drawn through the other. The difference in frequencies between the two oscillators is related to the concentration of the unknown gas. The actual frequencies are detected by pressure transducers, and the signals are processed electronically. Processed signals may be displayed via meters as percent concentrations or may be used as inputs to system control circuitry. Oscillator sensors currently have the capability to continuously measure the concentration of one gas. However, the use of multiple sen-

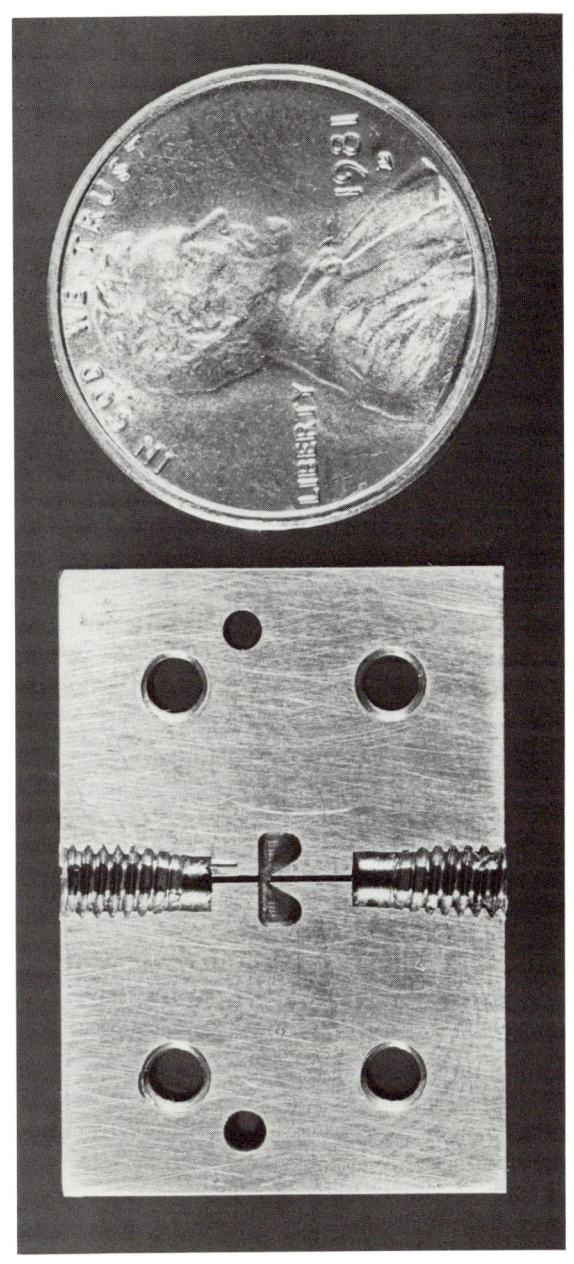

Figure 1. Jet-edge resonator oscillator with cover removed is shown beside a penny, illustrating its small size. (From Calkins, JM, et al[2] with permission.)

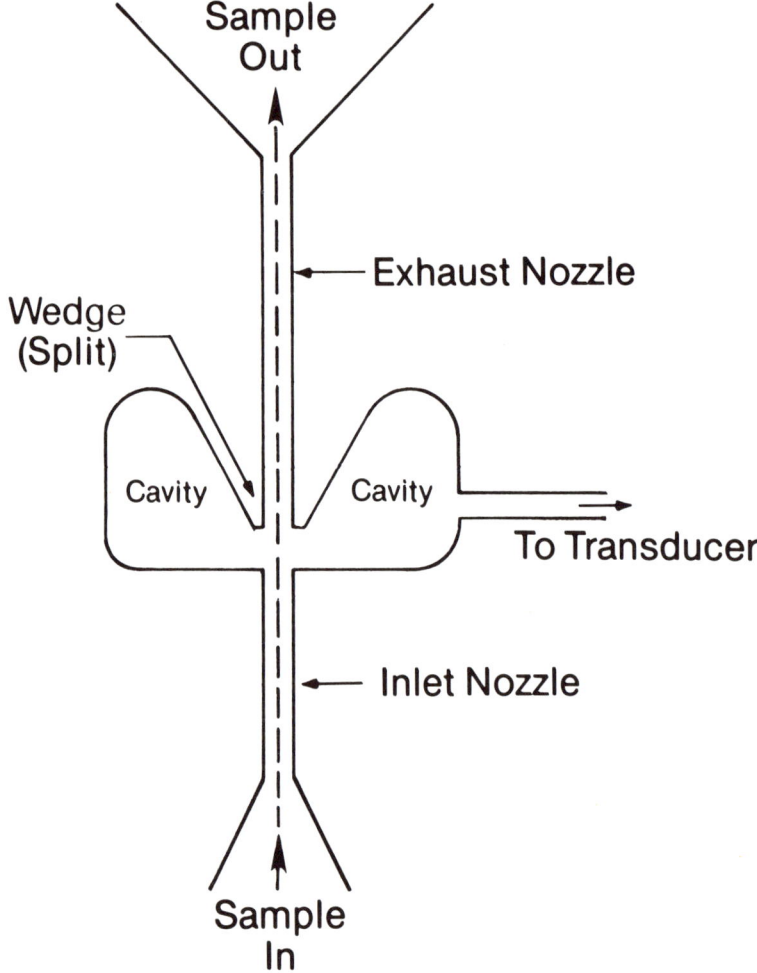

Figure 2. A schematic drawing of the flueric jet-edge resonator oscillator shows that this device consists of the jet edge (wedge), which is split to allow gas to exhaust and is surrounded by two resonating cavities. For a constant geometry, temperature, sample flow rate, and composition, the resulting frequency is produced by coupling of the jet edge with resonating cavity oscillations. (From Calkins, JM, et al,[2] with permission.)

sors of differing geometries will permit simultaneous multiple gas analyses. The change in frequency of the sensing unit is nearly linear with respect to the gas concentration. Time response for the sensor is adequate to permit detection of end-tidal and inspiratory peaks on a breath-by-breath basis.

Although jet-edge oscillators are not specific for a particular gas, they do measure gas concentrations accurately as long as binary or pseudobinary gas mixtures are presented. Accuracy is better than $\pm$ 1 percent, compared with infrared analyzers and standard gas mixtures. Flueric oscillators are temperature dependent and require temperature compensation but draw as little as 50 ml per minute of sample gas. Samples may be returned after analysis to the anesthetic circuit, if this is required for closed-circuit techniques.

Linear Resistor-Orifice Sensor (LROS)

Another fluidic sensor is the passive linear resistor-orifice sensor (LROS). It consists of a linear resistor and an orifice connected in series (Fig. 3). The LROS takes advantage of the differences in viscosity and density between gases, producing an analog differential pressure that is directly proportional to gas concentration. A further advantage is compact size and a low flow rate requirement. A differential pressure transducer is used to measure pressure drop across the device.

Both engineering and animal research evaluations of a prototype of this sensor system have been conducted. Engineering evaluation determined system linearity, sensitivity, time response, stability, and accuracy to be adequate for clinical applicability.

Electromechanical Anesthetic Monitor

An electromechanical volatile anesthetic monitor developed at the University of Arizona may be employed as a module in the Arizona system.[3,4] The device, which is placed in the anesthetic reservoir circuit, measures dimensional changes induced in a silicone polymer membrane by exposure to halogenated agents (Fig. 4 and Fig. 5). Dimensional changes in the membrane are measured by a linear variable differential transducer (LVDT), the core of which is resting on the center of the membrane. Data output from the device is via digital display and electrical signals in binary-coded decimal format. Setup of the device is accomplished by electromechanical zeroing and cali-

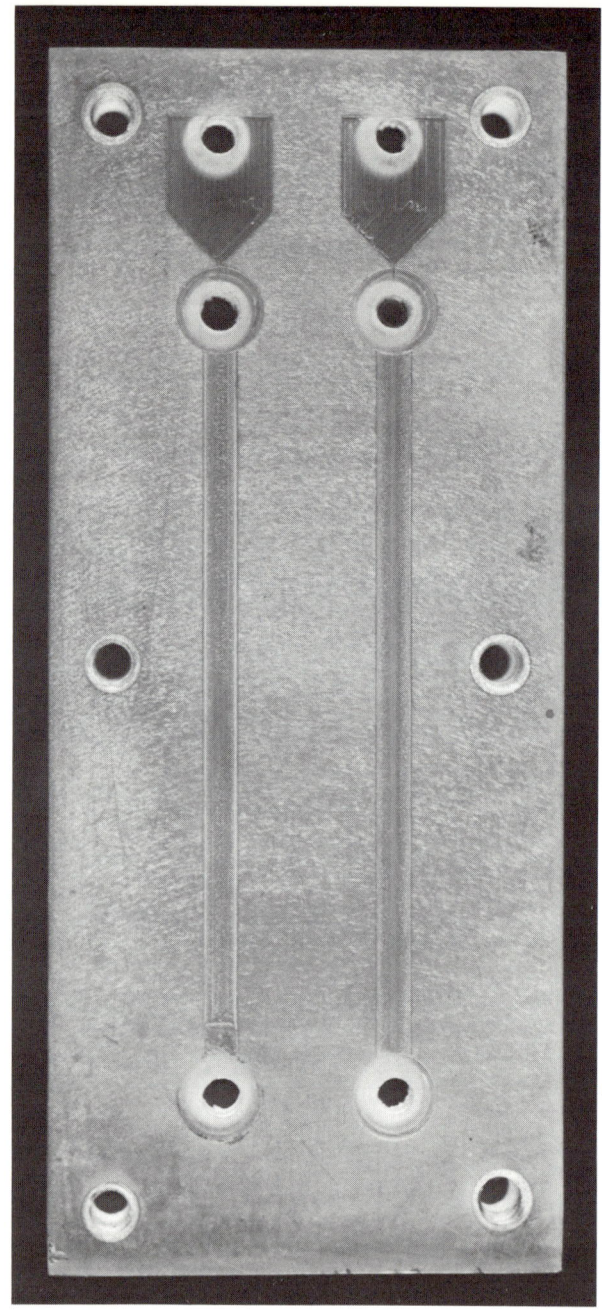

Figure 3. This is a linear resistor-orifice sensor (LROS) with the cover removed. Linear resistor channels are in series with fixed orifices (at point of V between ports). (From Calkins, JM, et al,[2] with permission.)

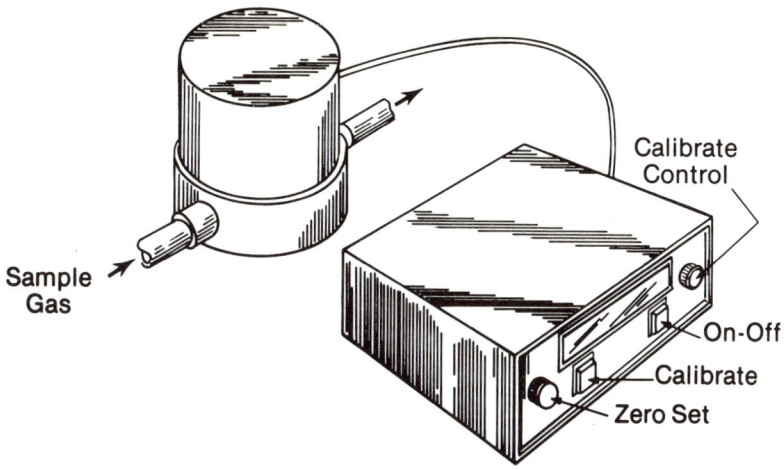

Figure 4. This illustration of the electromechanical anesthesia monitor shows the detector and calibration/display module.

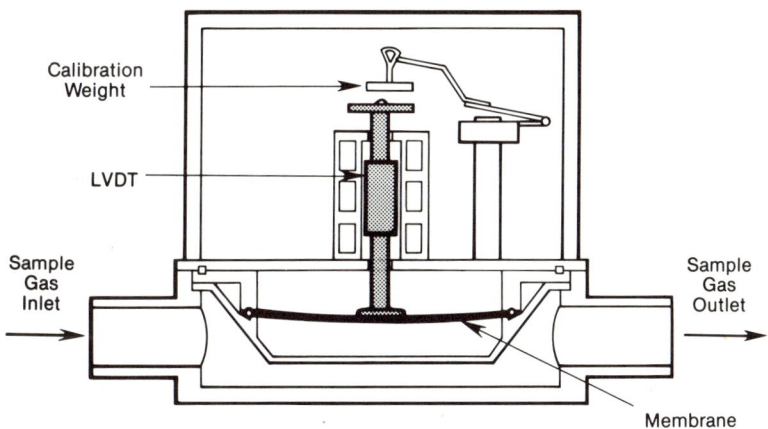

Figure 5. This is a cross-sectional view of the detector assembly of an anesthesia monitor. A linear variable differential transducer (LVDT) measures displacement of the membrane owing to anesthetic agents. A solenoid actuated weight dropped on the LVDT armature displaces the membrane by an amount equal to a known concentration for each anesthetic agent, providing a simple means of calibration.

bration: Zeroing involves a simple offset adjustment that facilitates use of the device with membranes of varying thicknesses; calibration is accomplished by dropping a standard weight onto the membrane and adjusting the gain appropriately. Deformation of the membrane owing to a fixed weight addition is equal to displacement caused by known anesthetic gas concentrations. The device is also compensated for variations in temperature and moisture. This device has been tested in the operating room, where satisfactory results were achieved. Over prolonged test periods using standardized gas mixtures, minimal drift occurred after initialization. Accuracy and reproducibility exceeded measurement capabilities of routine operating room equipment.

When combinations of volatile anesthetic and nitrous oxide are used, the total reading is more closely related to minimum alveolar concentration (MAC) than to concentration of volatile agent alone. Because MAC fractions are additive among anesthetic agents, it is believed that the device, in its present configuration, is best suited for use as a MAC monitor. It has been demonstrated that such an instrument or pair of instruments, fitted with two membranes of different silicone formulations, can provide discriminative single-agent measurements by differentiation of the volatile anesthetic and nitrous oxide. Time response provides average expired concentration.

Flow Sensors

The study of Saunders and coworkers[5] indicates the magnitude of inaccuracies to be found in lower flow rotameters (15 percent to 50 percent). Among the most accurate flowmeters adaptable for use in anesthesia machines is the linear resistance laminar flowmeter (LRLF). The LRLF measures gas flow through a rectangular channel in which flow is laminar over a given distance and over a defined range of flow rates. The pressure differential across a standard distance in the laminar flow path is linearly proportional to the flow rate. The device accuracy is better than 1 percent of full scale, measured against flowmeters having accuracy traceable to the National Bureau of Standards. Pressure can be measured visually, using differential pressure meters, and electronically, using differential pressure transducers. The ability to measure the flow electronically can provide microprocessor input, which in turn may regulate digital solenoid valve control of gas flow rates and concentrations. In addition, the LRLF has no moving parts and is easily disassembled for cleaning.

Several types of flowmeters, including disposable pneumotachometers, have been evaluated for respiratory flow measurement in the anesthesia circuit. These instruments are worthy of consideration for use in the system. Another type of flow measuring device which has been of particular value in high-frequency jet ventilation is the pitot tube. Advantages of this flow device include extremely fast response time and negligible flow resistance. Although pressure is not linear with flow, inclusion of a microprocessor allows accurate quantification of flow at virtually any rate and provides for real-time display of respiratory breath patterns. The pitot tube coupled to a solid-state pressure transducer is another candidate for inclusion in anesthesia delivery systems.

Physiologic Sensors

Input of physiologic data from the patient to the microprocessor of an automated anesthesia delivery system adds valuable dimensions to control and information systems. Algorithms utilizing blood gas, ECG, blood pressure, and other signals in conjunction with anesthesia uptake monitoring can provide the anesthesiologist with trend plots and facilitate crisis management.

ION SPECIFIC FIELD EFFECT TRANSISTORS (ISFETS)

In cooperation with the microelectronics laboratory of the University of Arizona, pH, electrolyte, and biochemical sensor development is underway. Numerous ion specific field effect transistors (ISFETS) have been fabricated and tested in vitro. To date, pH electrodes have remained accurate to ± 0.05 pH units in continuous measurements over a period of 18 months. ISFET membrane technology for sodium, calcium, potassium, and other substances is progressing slowly; their viability in use is presently only a matter of days or weeks. Because of their small size, however, these devices ultimately may be practical for continuous in vivo monitoring.

ESOPHAGEAL AND ENDOTRACHEAL MULTIPROBES

Electrocardiograph (ECG) monitoring in the operating room, a mainstay of patient care, is highly dependent upon the quality of the patient–instrument interface, that is, electrodes and leads. This is particularly true when monitoring the pediatric patient weighing less than 10 kg. Size of patient, surgical site, and so forth complicate electrode placement. A similar problem is frequently encountered in trauma or burn patients when electrode sites may be unavailable.

The development of endotracheal tubes incorporating electrocardiograph electrodes coupled via a high-gain isolation amplifier to an electrocardiograph monitor has shown evidence of providing a viable alternative to conventional attachment.[6] In the smaller-diameter endotracheal tubes, there is a possibility of embedding the conductive pathways in the tubing wall so as to avoid reduction of lumen size.

An esophageal multiprobe[7,8] using much of the same technology has also been extensively evaluated. This device, in addition to electrocardiograph signals, provides both heart-lung sounds and body core temperature. Coextruded conductive stripes embedded in the tubing wall permit flexibility without obstruction of the sound path.

BLOOD PRESSURE

An early, and somewhat unrelated, development by a member of the Anesthesia Research Group was a small apparatus for noninvasive measurement of blood pressure in dogs. As this device came to be used routinely in animal experimentation, the potential for use on pediatric patients undergoing surgery was explored. Minor electronic modification made the canine blood pressure instrument a convenient device for this application (Fig. 6). In the operating room, size, convenience, and ability to trend-monitor pressure changes are of primary importance to the anesthesiologist.

Recently, further refinement and circuitry additions have resulted in a microprocessor version of the original device which provides digital displays of systolic, diastolic, and mean pressures; heart rate; and pressure pulse product.[8] The complete system remains a hand-held instrument, the compactness of which affords particular value in neonatal and pediatric surgery.

CENTRAL NERVOUS SYSTEM (CNS) MONITORING

Inasmuch as sedation, analgesia, and to some extent muscle relaxation are related to central nervous system (CNS) activity, routine monitoring of cerebral function may enable the anesthetist to determine depth of anesthesia.

Central nervous system monitoring techniques are under study to assess the value of monitoring cerebral function as an indicator in anesthetic management. Because of complexity, inconsistency, and variability, the full lead electroencephalograph is not easily adapted for routine operating room use. However, with the development of

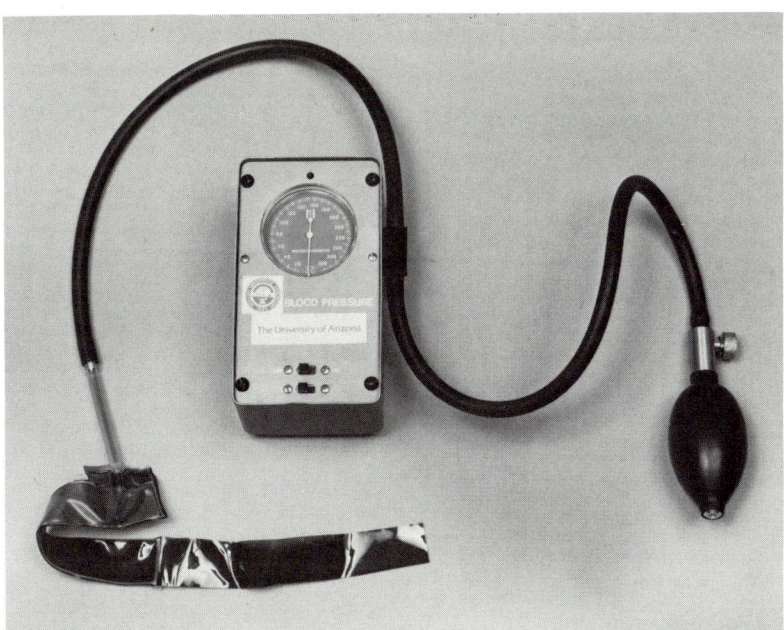

Figure 6. This is a photograph of a pediatric blood pressure instrument. A light-emitting diode above the pressure gauge turns on at systole, off at diastole. The special disposable 2 cm vinyl cuff attached is for neonatal use.

microelectronics, current technology makes passable devices that can translate the electroencephalogram into meaningful data. The Anesthesia Research Group is investigating several of these computer-assisted "simplified" electroencephalograph techniques.

The simplest of these is the two parameter electroencephalograph, also known as a cerebral function monitor (CFM). These devices electronically convert the complicated EEG into an average frequency and amplitude. The two parameter devices evolved from the need to present the anesthesiologist with an easily interpretable display. Unfortunately, sufficient clinical experience has not yet been gained to clearly assess the sensitivity and efficacy of this technique.

The next level of sophistication in cerebral monitoring with the electroencephalograph is the compressed spectral array (CSA). The utility of these devices is predicated on the pattern recognition ability of the anesthesiologist and contains more information about the electroencephalogram than the two parameter devices. The Arizona Group has developed its own Dot Spectral Array (DSA) system, which is a form of the CSA.

Although both approaches have been used successfully to detect severe compromise of cerebral perfusion, no clinical study has yet been performed to compare the sensitivities of these two techniques to hypoxia, depth of anesthesia, or other dependent variables such as blood pressure and choice of anesthetic agent.

Electromyogram (EMG) (derived from the forehead) is also under investigation as a potential indicator of anesthetic depth. Forehead EMG reflects CNS status by showing predictable changes associated with anesthesia. Monitoring this parameter may be considered a quantification of frowning or grimacing (used subjectively by clinicians) and, as such, may preferentially reflect the analgesic aspect of anesthesia.

DELIVERY OF ANESTHETIC AGENTS

Automation of anesthesia delivery is clearly the direction of the future. Automation will include new high-technology components with improved economics, self-surveillance, and predictability. The Arizona concept of such an apparatus, with the necessary subsystems and components previously discussed, is diagrammed in Figure 7. Components include 1) gas supply and proportioning; 2) volatile anesthetic delivery; 3) the breathing circuit, complete with scavenging, humidification, and carbon dioxide absorbers; 4) sensors; 5) ventilator; 6) the computer, with appropriate inputs and outputs for integration into the machine-anesthesiologist-patient relationship.

Gas Proportionating System

The gas proportionating system of Figure 8 is applicable to both automated and manual modes of anesthesia delivery. This apparatus is being designed to meet the following operational criteria:

1. Total flow rate
   High flow—1 liter per minute to 10 liters per minute $\pm$ 0.25 liter per minute
   Low flow (closed circuit)—50 ml per minute to 1 liter per minute $\pm$ 10 ml per minute
2. Nitrous oxide concentration—0 percent to 70 percent $\pm$ 2 percent

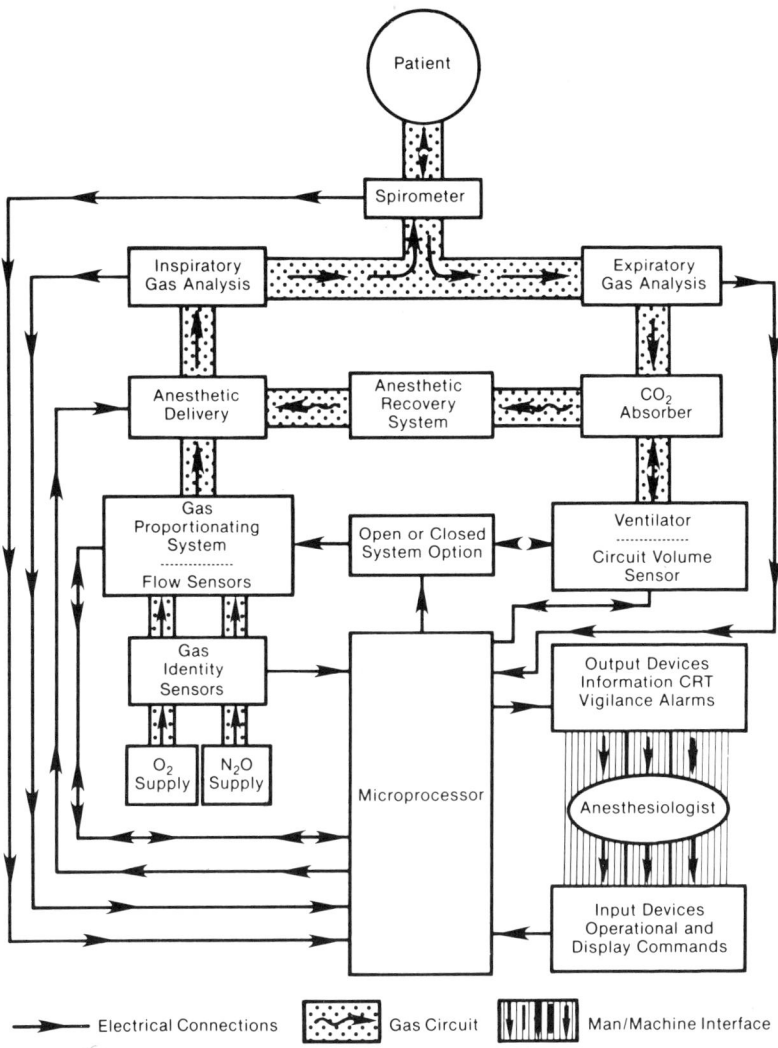

Figure 7. This is a schematic drawing of the Arizona anesthesia delivery system.

3. Neither total flow rate nor nitrous oxide concentration will vary more than the specified error margin for a pressure variation at the breathing mask of −10 cm water to 60 cm water.
4. Oxygen concentrations of less than 30 percent delivered to the circuit should not be possible. (Of course, the circuit can still

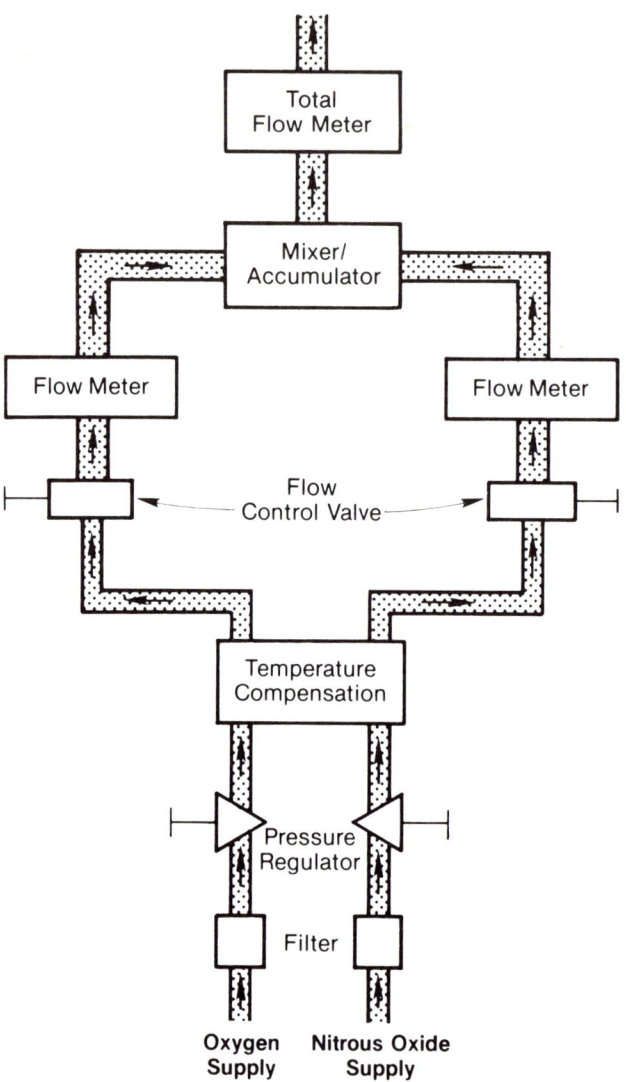

Figure 8. This is a schematic drawing of a gas proportionating system.

provide a hypoxic inspired mixture to the patient, so expired oxygen monitoring is mandatory as usual.)

Several configurations and component choices are being considered for use in the proportionator module. The following elements have been evaluated:

1. Linear resistance laminar flowmeters (LRLF) were coupled to solid-state differential pressure transducers to provide an analog voltage proportional to flow. This output is available for numeric display and controller input.

2. Fixed orifice valves with positive solenoid open-close drives were used to regulate flow. An electronic control mechanism or the anesthesia system microprocessor maintains the desired flow by adjusting the frequency and duration of valve "on" time. Feedback from the flowmeters provides nearly instantaneous correction, and back pressure and temperature effects are eliminated. The rugged structure, reliability, and ease of servicing of the components within the proportionating module offer important advantages in both high-flow and closed-circuit anesthesia.

Volatile Anesthetic Delivery

Fluidic atomizers, solenoid injectors, and other means of introduction of volatile anesthetic agents into the breathing circuit have been considered for inclusion in the Arizona System. All these methods appear to be reliable. The simplest technique, however, may be a syringe servo pump driven by a stepping motor responsive to microprocessor digital signals.

In tests, the syringe pump has been used to inject anesthetic agents onto stainless steel mesh within a T piece in the recirculating expiratory gas stream. Preliminary data indicate that halothane concentrations from this pump delivery can be maintained within ± 0.03 percent.

A safety feature and future design element is encodement for anesthetic agent and volume by means of container size or shape. A receiver portion of the pump mechanism will transmit the container code via contact switches to microprocessor or controller. This signal, in conjunction with inspiratory gas sensors, will provide redundant sources for administered anesthetic identity.

Volatile Anesthetic Recovery

Recovery of volatile anesthetic agents by condensation has been investigated as an alternative to present scavenger and exhaust techniques. Originally, it was felt that by means of cold condensation, volatile anesthetic returned to the liquid state might be reused. This could be of particular economic importance in open-circuit, high-flow anesthesia. Separation of the volatile agent from water vapor and other compounds may present a problem, as does the possible degradation of halothane by soda lime in the carbon dioxide absorber. Reduction of atmospheric pollution remains a potential impetus for adapting such a procedure.

One of the proposed recovery systems employs staged vortex tubes, a gas-powered device through which inspiratory gases pass en route to the patient. One end of the vortex tube, the "hot side," is used as a vaporizer; the other end, the "cold junction," drives a condenser in the breathing circuit. Condensate of the volatile agent is retained in a baffled reservoir, where it is prevented from re-entering the circuit.

Ventilators

One of the most important modules in any anesthesia delivery system is the ventilator. Research within the Arizona Group has been directed to the creation of guidelines for the design of a standard anesthesia ventilator as well as development of pediatric and high-frequency jet ventilators. Enumerated in Table 1 are the functions to be incorporated in an anesthesia ventilator.

Table 1. Design Guidelines for a Standard Anesthesia Ventilator

A. Controls should regulate the ventilator in such a manner that whether operated manually or set by microprocessor, device parameters are keyed to patient physiologic function.
B. Controls should be noninteractive, and adjustment of rate, I/E ratio, and tidal or minute volume must be totally independent.
C. The anesthesia ventilator should operate in either open- or closed-circuit modes. Closed-circuit use further requires that accurate means are incorporated for determination of respiratory and circuit volumes.
D. The device should be applicable to pediatric anesthesia, with high precision both in control and in accuracy.
E. PEEP and humidification control should be incorporated into the instrument.
F. Means should be provided, either as part of the ventilator or in conjunction with it, for data collection on machine function and for patient records.
G. Numerically scaled analog controls that are easily seen and adjusted by the anesthesiologist should be placed in a convenient location.
H. Transducers to provide information about status and performance to the microprocessor or other control means should also be incorporated.
I. Finally, it is desirable to provide an instrument of the smallest possible size because of space constraints.

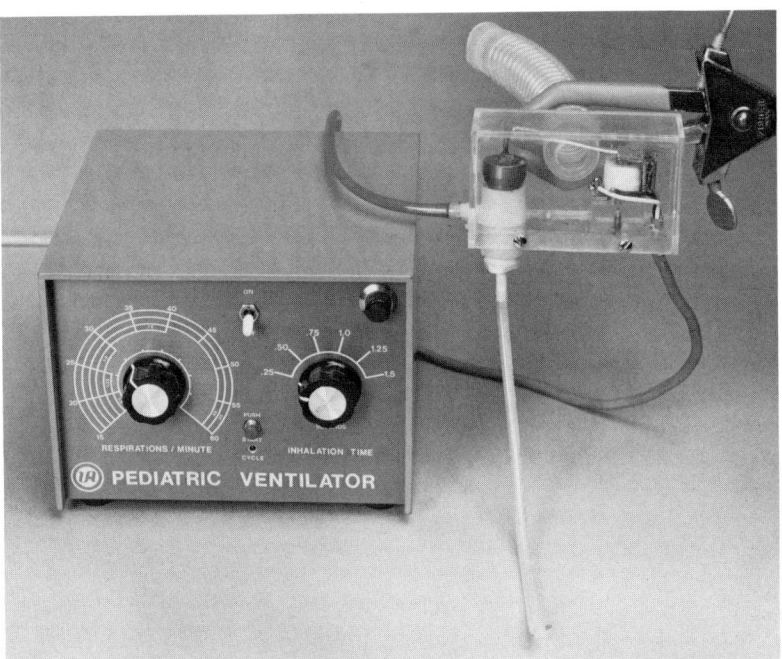

Figure 9. This is a photograph of the Arizona pediatric ventilator. The valve-actuating mechanism is shown on the right, with endotracheal tube attached.

PEDIATRIC ANESTHESIA VENTILATOR

A very simple pediatric anesthesia ventilator has been constructed and tested on animals. Its primary advantage is an exceedingly small dead space volume (Fig. 9). This device consists of a timing circuit providing respiratory frequencies of 15 to 60 cpm and inhalation times of 0.25 to 1.5 seconds. Mounted in a manifold immediately adjacent to the patient airway is an operations solenoid driven by the solid-state timer. This solenoid displaces a valving plug on one arm of a T piece. The weight of the plug can be adjusted over the range of 30 to 60 cm water to permit blowoff in case of overpressurization. The exhalation limb of the manifold will accommodate a PEEP valve. Simplicity and reliability make this inexpensive instrument ideal for use in small animal research as well as pediatric applications.

HIGH-FREQUENCY VENTILATORS

Investigations into high-frequency ventilation and its extension into new techniques of anesthesia delivery are presently under way.[10-15]

Areas of interest include instrumentation of high-frequency systems in order to quantify their input characteristics; defining operational variables and their relationship to physiologic effects; examining the homeostatic impact of high-frequency ventilation on the organism as a whole; comparisons of high-frequency jet (HFJV) with high-frequency oscillatory ventilation (HFOV) techniques for efficacy; development of mechanical analogs of lung and airways to better understand the mechanisms of gas exchange with both HFJV and HFOV.

It has become obvious that high-frequency ventilation techniques are efficacious in obtaining a particular blood gas but may cause other chemical and metabolic disturbances, the mechanisms of which are not yet understood. Studies are aimed at the identification of those areas outside of present use for otolaryngology and routine ventilatory support where high-frequency ventilation may be of particular value in the operating suite.

CONTROL OF ANESTHESIA DELIVERY

Incorporation of the microprocessor into future anesthesia machines for monitoring and control has brought about a great deal of research into modes of data acquisition and processing. A computer-based system has been created, providing breath-by-breath information, trend analysis, and anesthetic status.[16] Real-time output parameters include absolute values and ratios of inspired and end-tidal anesthetic concentrations, inspired and expired tidal volumes, single-breath and cumulative anesthetic uptake, the elapsed time and square root of time of anesthesia delivery, respiratory rate, and apnea detection. This system is noninvasive, requiring only two continuous inputs: patient respiratory flow and anesthetic concentration in respiratory gases. Results of laboratory simulation methods applied to system functions indicate that accuracy and reproducibility are well within the tolerance of commonly used clinical devices.

Animal studies have been conducted on a microprocessor-controlled closed loop anesthesia delivery system.[17] The user enters, via the processor keyboard, the desired patient concentration of anesthetic, patient weight, and the total volume of the system. The Arizona anesthesia electromechanical monitor (described elsewhere) provides the exhaled anesthetic concentration. The program calculates and displays the time and dose of anesthetic to be delivered. Estimated cardiac output, total time, and cumulative anesthetic dose are also displayed. Although this study was directed toward evaluation of a monitor-responsive control system, it may be seen that the microprocessor output could be used to directly regulate anesthetic introduction into the closed loop.

SUMMARY

Research by the Advanced Biotechnology Group, Department of Anesthesiology, the University of Arizona, has led to the development of many of the physical and theoretic elements necessary to the creation of a new automated anesthesia delivery system. Recognizing the obligation to provide means of the highest reliability and safety for anesthesia delivery, this group is endeavoring to bring together a compact, integrated modular system of the greatest utility to the practicing anesthesiologist.

REFERENCES

1. MYLREA, KC, ET AL: *Automated Anesthesia Delivery and Patient Management in the Operating Room.* In KARIN, S (ED): *24th Midwest Symposium on Circuits and Systems.* University of New Mexico, 1981.
2. CALKINS, JM, ET AL: *A flueric respiratory and anesthetic gas analyzer.* Annals of Biomedical Engineering, vol. 10, number 2, 1982, pp. 83–96.
3. CALKINS, JM, ET AL: *A new electromechanical anesthesia monitor.* IEEE 1980 Frontiers of Engineering in Health Care, 1980, pp 101–104.
4. JEWETT, WR, ET AL: United States Patent 4,150,670.
5. SAUNDERS, RJ, CALKINS, JM, GOODEN, TM: *Accuracy in rotameters and linear flowmeters.* Annual Meeting, American Society of Anesthesiologists, October, 1981. Anesthesiology (Suppl) 55:3A, p 116.
6. MYLREA, KC, ET AL: *An EKG lead with the endotracheal tube.* Critical Care Medicine, March, 1983.
7. MYLREA, KC, ET AL: United States Patent 4,176,660.
8. DEMER, JL, ET AL: *An esophageal multiprobe for temperature, electrocardiogram and heart and lung sounds measurements.* IEEE Transactions on Biomedical Engineering vol 25:4, 1978, p 377.
9. JEWETT, WR: United States Patent 4,290,434.
10. CALKINS, JM, *A Simple Flueric High Frequency Jet Ventilator,* Anesth Analg (Cleve) 61:2, 1982, pp 138–141.
11. CALKINS, JM, ET AL: *Jet pulse characteristics for high frequency jet ventilation in dogs.* Anesth Analg (Cleve) 61:2, 1982, pp 293–300.
12. WATERSON, CK, ET AL: *High frequency jet ventilation operational guidelines.* Anesth Analg (Cleve) 61:2, 1982, p 222.

13. QUAN, SF, ET AL: *High frequency ventilation—a promising new method of ventilation.* Heart Lung vol. 12, number 2, March, 1983, pp 152–155.
14. WATERSON, CK AND CALKINS, JM: *Mechanical Analog for High Frequency Ventilation.* Proceedings 17th Annual Meeting, AAMI, May, 1982.
15. OTTO, CW, ET AL: *Hemodynamic effects of high frequency jet ventilation.* Anesth Analg (Cleve) 62:298–304, 1983.
16. LAURIA, MJ, ET AL: A real time anesthesia data acquisition and processing system. IEEE Transactions, Biomedical Engineering 29:8, 1982, p 604.
17. MYLREA, KC, ET AL: *Closed loop anesthesia delivery under microprocessor control.* 15th Annual Meeting AAMI, 1980, p 148.

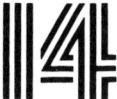

THE BOSTON ANESTHESIA SYSTEM

Jeffrey B. Cooper, Ph.D., and
Ronald S. Newbower, Ph.D.

The conventional anesthesia machine is a mechanically reliable medical device. Unfortunately, in the routine clinical environment, it is, at best, an awkward piece of equipment supporting an array of gadgets which surround the user and compete with the patient for attention. Moreover, machine data are not presented to the anesthesiologist in a simple absorbable form and cannot be directly captured, transmitted, or analyzed by peripheral electronic devices. The sheer size and inflexibility of the machine and its complement of displays is a frustration to the human-factors expert. The net effect is to encourage the commission of error in its use.

Approximately 10 years ago, we began a study of these problems and of ways to overcome them through creative use of current technology, particularly state-of-the-art electronics. The resulting prototype was dubbed the Boston Anesthesia System (BAS)—an electronically based anesthesia delivery system.[1] It was intended to catalyze fresh thinking in the technologist's approach to anesthesia problems and to demonstrate the potential of an integrated design.

To support the design effort, we undertook an elaborate multihospital study of preventable mishaps in anesthesia in order to analyze the role devices play in allowing or encouraging human error.[2,3,4] After careful analysis of 790 preventable mishaps in four hospitals, we concluded that approximately 89 percent were attributable to human error. Only 11 percent could be attributed to mechanical failures. In addition, only a small percentage of those mechanical failures were traceable to malfunctions of an anesthesia machine. They do, indeed, appear to be mechanically reliable.

However, approximately one third of the human errors were involved in an interaction with the anesthesia machine or its associated breathing circuit. The implication was strong that attention was due to the interface of human practitioners with their instrumentation.

Figure 1 is an aid in considering these issues. It is a schematic representation of the interdependent relationships between the equipment, anesthetist, and patient. In managing patients, some measurement of status is made, using the anesthesiologist's own senses, including technologic extensions of those senses. Decisions and actions are made and carried out using the anesthesia delivery system, which includes the machine, intravenous apparatus, ventilators, and so forth. The performance of any given system must be monitored by the anesthetist as closely as the status of the anesthetized patient.

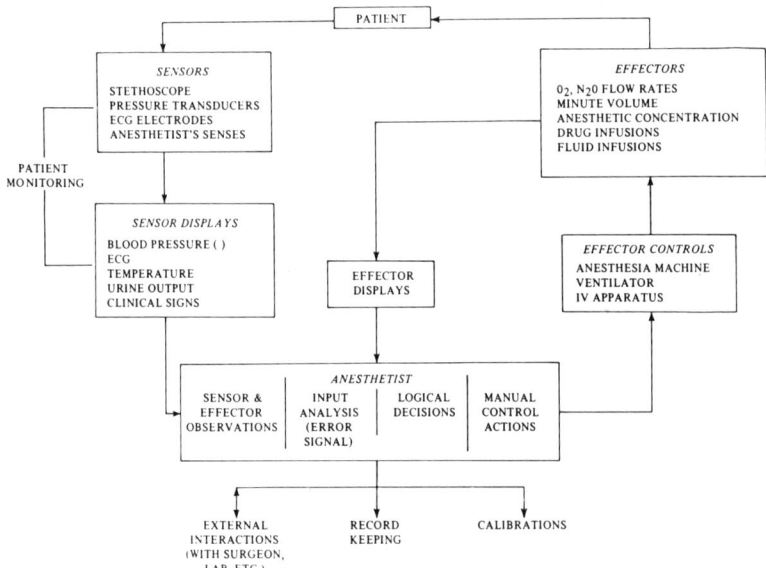

Figure 1. This is a schematic representation of the anesthesia management system. (From Cooper, JB: *Anesthesia management systems*. In Gravenstein, JS, ET AL: *Monitoring Surgical Patients in the Operating Room*. Charles C Thomas, Springfield, IL, 1979, with permission.)

Technologic aids must be reliable, rugged, fail safe, and effective. Yet the operating room environment is very hostile to devices and apparatus. The machine–man communication link is critical in the system and must function effectively with minimal attention and effort. The flow of information around the loop must be constant and accurate to support safe care.

These various constraints and requirements served as guidelines for us in the selection of technologic strategies for a fresh approach to the design of an improved anesthesia delivery system. To this end, we have designed, fabricated, and tested the BAS prototype. It can serve as a reference point for discussions for another anesthesia system and for the role that technology must play in anesthesia care. To aid in that process, we will describe some of the rationale of our approach and the choices we made.

PROTOTYPE DESIGN AND FUNCTION

In order to design and to fabricate successfully an apparatus that will meet the constraints previously described, it has become clear that a substantial amount of electronic technology must be involved. Sensing gases, organizing information, keeping records, and implementing alarms are all functions that require electronic technology for flexibility, effectiveness, and efficiency. Unfortunately, hybrid systems involving marriages of new electronic technology with traditional mechanical technology are complex and cumbersome. For example, the simple attachment of servo motors to needle valves is not an appealing technologic approach for flow control. We concluded at the outset of our efforts that it was necessary to acquire or to develop methods of metering gas flows and liquid anesthetics that are inherently compatible with electronic technologies and control. This would enable the development to be reasonably simple, coherent, and reliable.

Our design is based entirely upon the use of on/off devices with few moving parts. No rotameters, servo motors, or potentiometers are used for control functions. Flow calibration depends on the tolerances of fixed orifices rather than of sliding parts. Sensors are used primarily as components for safety checks and for monitoring critical functions of the system. No flow sensors are used for control.

The general structure of our prototype is shown schematically in Figure 2. The desired mixtures of oxygen and nitrous oxide are generated by special digital valves. Volatile anesthetics are added

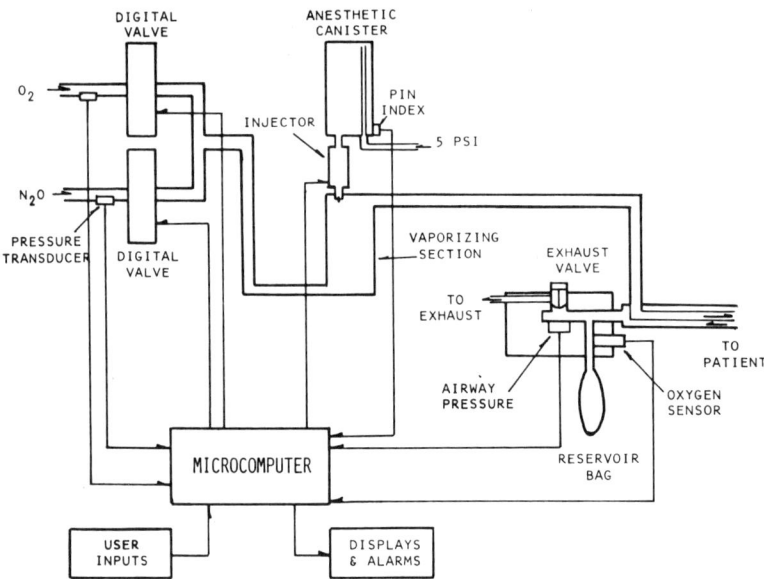

Figure 2. This is a schematic representation of the prototype anesthesia machine. The term microcomputer refers to the ensemble of the microprocessor with its necessary support electronics. (From Cooper, JB, et al,[1] with permission.)

directly into the gas mixture in pulses by an injection device. The injected liquid vaporizes in a passive evaporator coil. The active devices are under the control of a microprocessor which receives instructions from the control panel and scans a number of other vital machine sensors. Anesthesia system function is continuously monitored by the processor, which either corrects or alarms when either the machine or the user acts inappropriately. The processor itself is separately monitored to insure appropriate action. Rechargeable batteries provide backup power in the event of electrical line failure. The state of charge of the batteries is one of the continuously monitored variables.

This simple prototype system performs the basic task of any conventional anesthesia machine, but by employing a microprocessor-based architecture it allows orderly expansion and communication with other electronic devices such as monitors and computers. It will accept new sensors relatively easily, while allowing development of practical automated record-keeping techniques. This technology also allows important innovations in the design of machine–man interfaces with the intent of reducing human error.

As shown in Figure 2, the prototype anesthesia delivery system consists of several subsystems that are appropriately linked and controlled via inputs and outputs from a microcomputer. These subsystems can be divided into those of gas proportioning, volatile anesthetic delivery, and microprocessor control, all delivering the appropriate mixture to the breathing circuit.

Gas Delivery Subsystem

The anesthetic gases, oxygen and nitrous oxide, are supplied from either yoke-mounted cylinders or standard pipeline connections. The pressures of these gases are reduced by standard regulators with filtering through separate line filters. Solid state pressure transducers monitor the pressure downstream of each filter for use by the controlling microprocessor.

The flow of each gas is controlled separately by an eight-element digital flow controller. Each of these controllers consists of a parallel group of calibrated orifices, the flow resistances of which are weighted in a binary fashion. Each subsequent open orifice delivers twice the flow of the one below it in the sequence. The control of flow through each orifice is accomplished by an associated solenoid valve. The array of orifices is directly controlled by a binary word from the microprocessor. The assembly is inherently digital and extremely reliable.

Flow rate does not depend on tolerances of any moving parts, as with conventional needle valves. Each orifice is actually designed as a sonic nozzle. Its shape is such that the speed of sound will occur in the throat of the nozzle when the pressure drop across the orifice exceeds 20 percent of the absolute upstream pressure. Under these conditions, the nozzle's flow is relatively independent of any downstream pressure fluctuations and can be accurately predicted from a knowledge of only the upstream pressure and the nozzle's fixed calibration. The microprocessor is programmed to perform the computations necessary to achieve the desired flow.

Volatile Anesthetic Subsystem

The gas flowing from the two digital valves is the appropriate mixture of oxygen and nitrous oxide. Liquid inhalation anesthetic is injected directly into that gas stream in boluses of approximately 5 microliters. The injector device is an automotive fuel injector slightly modified to improve its resistance to deterioration from exposure to various anesthetic agents. It is a solenoid operated on/off valve. The pulse time width and liquid driving pressure are maintained at constant values. Hence, the injected liquid volume varies only with the physical properties of the liquid. A calibration factor for each anesthetic is permanently stored in the machine's memory and used in the appropriate electronic processing.

The necessary frequency of injector pulses is calculated by the processor according to its stored program. The frequency is a function of the selected total gas flow rate, the desired concentration of anesthetic, the calibration factor involved, and a known ratio of liquid volume to vapor volume at standard temperature and pressure. The liquid is atomized into a chamber as it emerges from the injector, and complete vaporization is easily achieved in a passive vaporizing coil. Temperature compensation is therefore not necessary.

A unique feature deriving from this system is a disposable or reusable canister that is magnetically coded to indicate which volatile liquid anesthetic is contained within. The canister is mounted in a socket in the table top of the work surface. A magnetic sensing device in the mounting area informs the microprocessor which canister is in place. Opportunities for mix-ups are greatly reduced. These canisters are made from a nylon polymer resistant to deterioration from volatile anesthetics.

Microprocessor Controller

The microprocessor in the prototype is an INTEL 8080.[5] The displays, digital valve, and injector are all operated by this microprocessor. It is a compact dedicated computer which is permanently programmed to perform the tasks of this particular anesthesia system. It is in the form of 12 circuit boards, which are in the base cabinet. These include a central processing unit, memory (8000 bytes), an analog-digital converter (16 channels), a sequencing clock, special circuits for input and output information (24 I/O ports), and a number of other special circuits. The controller performs several major tasks which have been, for convenience, divided into communication functions and control functions.

The communication functions include 1) interpretation of commands from console switches, 2) displaying current measured values and control settings, and 3) displaying alarms for unsafe or inappropriate conditions resulting from various types of error. The control functions include 1) reading sensors, 2) computing effector settings from operator commands and sensor readings, and 3) setting effectors.

Each specific task is described by a programmed sequence of steps contained in permanent memory. The entire program is executed every second. During one program cycle, one subroutine may be repeated several times, but the user has no specific perception that this repetitive computing is occurring. The machine will respond quickly to any command.

The processor is programmed to operate in a fail-safe manner. For example, when oxygen supply pressure decreases to lower than normal range, the processor resets the digital valve to continue to deliver the same gas flow while displaying an alarm message. When the oxygen pressure becomes totally inadequate, all flows are terminated and an additional loud alarm is sounded to indicate that this event has occurred.

Inasmuch as a fundamental characteristic of the programmed controller is flexibility, major changes in the method of operation for the entire prototype system are easily and quickly completed. Changes involve rewriting the program and loading this modified program into the memory devices. Programmable read-only memories are used for permanent storage in the prototype machine. Similarly, a manufactured version of this system could be modified to meet specific needs. Modifications must, of course, be carefully considered, lest they undermine the previously refined, safe, and effective performance of the system. The core program need not and should not be modified for specific user applications.

Breathing Circuit

The complete system is designed to enable the use of low-flow as well as high-flow anesthetic techniques. The accuracies of the metering devices as well as the resolution of the controls and displays were determined with that in mind. However, for preliminary trials and demonstrations, we arbitrarily chose to design and to construct a relatively simple breathing circuit without carbon dioxide absorption based on the Bain circuit. An oxygen sensor and airway pressure sensor are installed internally. An adjustable exhaust (pop-off) valve sends excessive gas through external piping to a reservoir chamber. This reservoir is continuously scavenged by direct connection to a standard suction line.

The oxygen sensor employed is a standard commercially available polarographic unit mounted in a modified prototype housing. The sensor monitors oxygen concentration at the outlet of the expiratory tube. This is an independent measurement which assists in verification of gas composition in the breathing circuit. The measured value (displayed on the console) is not used for gas flow control. A low oxygen value activates an alarm message. Failure of this electrochemical sensor does not compromise any other aspect of system performance.

Operation of the Prototype

The prototype of the Boston Anesthesia System is shown in Figure 3. The upper console is the control unit. All necessary information has been organized on this panel. Controls and displays of machine function are grouped on the left side (Fig. 4). The right side of the console contains a message panel for displaying warnings and alarms. Future expansion could include display of electronically generated trend analysis and any anesthetic record information desired.

Flows and concentrations are indicated by illuminated bar graph columns (see Figure 4). Each column is color coded with an illuminated scale alongside. Settings are changed by operating the color-coded (increment/decrement) switches located below each bar label. The left-hand bar represents total gas flow, ranging from 0 to 10 liters per minute. The second bar indicates nitrous oxide concentration in volume percent. It is adjustable in concentrations from 0 to 100 percent with certain time restrictions on operation above 80 percent. The third column is automatically labelled with the name of the volatile anesthetic put into the machine via the coded canisters. The remaining columns display measured values of expired oxygen concentration and airway pressure and have no associated control switches. The system can be operated in either a conventional format (that is, individual oxygen and nitrous oxide flow controls) or an alternative mode in which total flow, percent nitrous oxide, and percent volatile anesthetic agent are the control variables. The latter technique represents a more physiologic basis for controlling the breathing mixture and may eliminate some of the errors associated with the use of individual rotameter controls.

Three push-button switches which are located on the lower portion of the console have special functions. One button enables the user to

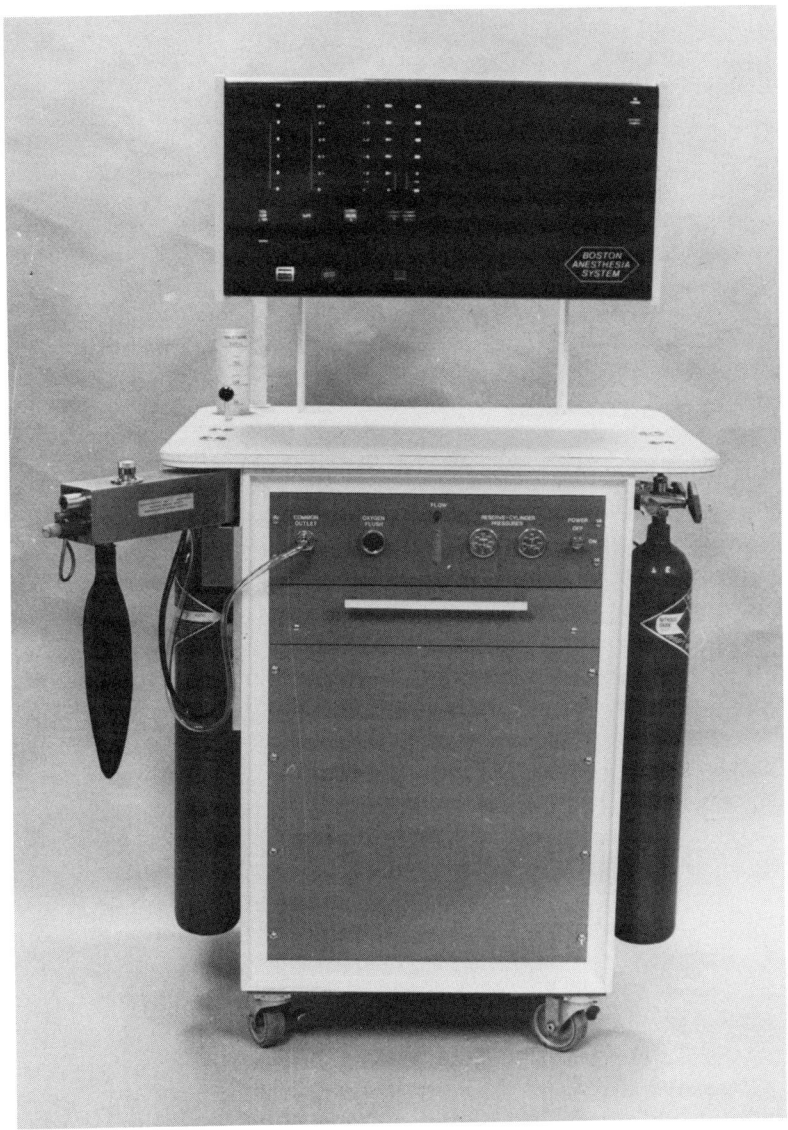

Figure 3. This is the Boston Anesthesia System. (From Cooper, JB, et al,[1] with permission.)

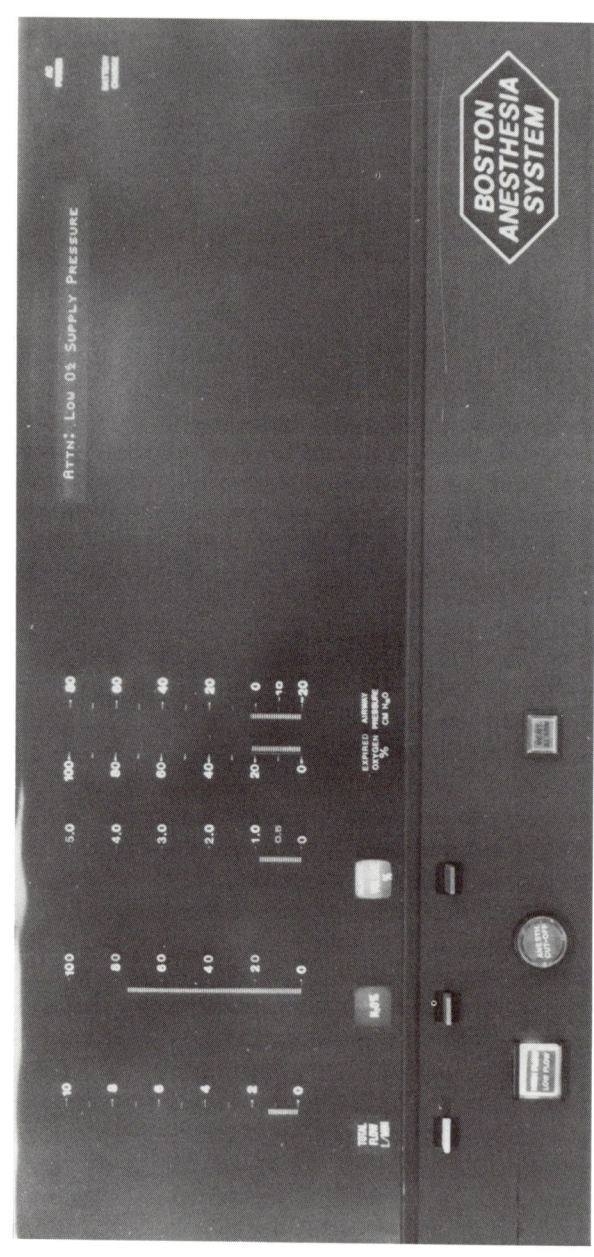

Figure 4. This is a close-up view of the Boston Anesthesia System operating console. The switch levers, bar labels, and scale markings are all color coded. The volatile anesthetic label indicates that a halothane canister was in use. An alarm message is being displayed. (From Cooper, JB, et al,[1] with permission.)

switch all the concentration displays from a high-flow range to a low-flow range affording improved resolution. The round button is an anesthetic cutoff switch. When this button is depressed, the flows of all anesthetics are unambiguously terminated. The third control push-button activates a ventilator alarm function in which airway pressure is automatically and continuously monitored in search of a ventilation cycle at least every 30 seconds. A breathing circuit disconnection or other failure to ventilate will result in an alarm message.

The compact control console is actually detachable from the large base of the machine. In theory, it could be moved to another location. Duplication in a slave console is immediately suggested and could be easily implemented for a wide variety of purposes. A small, roughly calibrated rotameter flowmeter is located in the center of the front panel at the base cabinet (see Figure 3). This flowmeter is provided to lend assurance to any skeptical user that gas is flowing properly. The power on/off switch, reserve cylinder pressure gauges, and oxygen flush control are located on the same panel. Oxygen flush is mechanically actuated, providing a backup for life support in the event of any major electronic failure.

Alarm Functions

The current system is capable of delivering 16 different warning messages. When an unsafe condition exists or an inappropriate action is attempted, the message is displayed in the upper right section of the console. A message is also accompanied by a distinctive audio alarm repeated every five seconds. The audio signals will attract the user's attention to the panel. When more than one problem exists at any given time, the message with the highest priority is displayed until the problem is corrected. Subsequent messages will appear in order until all problems are resolved. The messages are designed in a self-explanatory manner. For instance, attempting to set a nitrous oxide concentration prior to choosing a nonzero value for the total gas flow is one of the conditions in which the message "Please Increase Total Gas Flow" would be displayed. The message "Attn: Hypoxic Gas Mixture" is displayed when the delivery oxygen concentration is set below 20 percent in any operating mode. The machine will allow such a condition to exist for as long as 45 seconds and will then automatically readjust flow ratio to create a 50 percent oxygen mixture. If a low oxygen concentration on the expiratory side of the breathing circuit exists, an additional alarm will sound.

The microprocessor performs a variety of checks on the operation of the system every 0.1 seconds. Hence, mechanical difficulties are reported with appropriate alarm messages. For example, a decrease in oxygen supply pressure leads automatically to display of "Attn: Low O_2 Supply Pressure." A low state of charge of backup battery power supply is also indicated by a message. The full array is presented in reference 1.

Development and Design Concept

A framework for integrating anesthesia monitoring and control has been created. Some previously impractical or cumbersome physiologic monitoring and record-keeping concepts can now be reexamined. Automated record keeping becomes more plausible, innovative clinical teaching methods suggest themselves, and studies of the anesthesia control loop may be facilitated. Technologies in this prototype were chosen with reliability and fail-safe operation as major criteria. The unit was designed to give overt indication of any difficulty and to revert to a safe mode in the event of any type of failure. Though only a prototype, the system has proven extremely reliable despite significant abuse encountered during shipment around the country for display and demonstration.

Still, we are keenly aware that replacement of the traditional anesthesia machine with an electronic system will introduce risks and unknowns. Acceptance by the anesthesia community will ultimately depend on positive experiences, an extensive history of clinical reliability, and the attainment of certain standards of safe performance. This can be accomplished only when production-engineered versions of such a system are readily available. We expect that it is only a matter of time until that is accomplished.

REFERENCES

1. COOPER, JB, NEWBOWER, RS, MOORE, JW, ET AL: *A new anesthesia delivery system.* Anesthesiology 49:310–318, 1978.
2. COOPER, JB, NEWBOWER, RS, LONG, CD, ET AL: *Preventable anesthesia mishaps—a human factors study.* Anesthesiology 49:399–406, 1978.
3. COOPER, JB, LONG, CD, NEWBOWER, RS: *Human error in anesthesia management.* In GRUNDY, BL AND GRAVENSTEIN, JS (EDS): *The Quality of Care in Anesthesia.* Charles C Thomas, Springfield, IL, 1982.

4. NEWBOWER, RS, COOPER, JB, AND LONG, CD: *Learning from anesthesia mishaps.* QRB 7:10–16, 1981.
5. TRAUTMAN, ED, COOPER, JB, AND NEWBOWER, RS: *A new anesthesia delivery system using microprocessors.* Proc IEEE Electro 76 Conference, Boston, 1976.

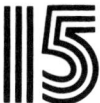

THE UTAH SYSTEM: COMPUTER-CONTROLLED ANESTHETIC DELIVERY

Dwayne R. Westenskow, Ph.D., and
William S. Jordan, M.D.

Traditional anesthesia machines provide a means for delivering desired flows of oxygen, nitrous oxide, and volatile anesthetic agents to the patient as well as a means for setting the tidal volume and respiratory rate for mechanical ventilation. These, however, are not the variables of greatest concern to the anesthetist. The goals during general anesthesia include achieving and maintaining a desired level of anesthesia by delivering appropriate anesthetic concentrations to the brain; delivering sufficient oxygen to the lung to provide adequate arterial oxygenation; and maintaining an appropriate arterial carbon dioxide concentration by appropriately adjusting ventilation. It is preferable that the anesthesia machine have adjustments for the brain concentrations of volatile anesthetics, arterial blood oxygen concentrations, and arterial carbon dioxide concentrations rather than controls of gas and vapor flow rates to the delivery system or tidal volume and respiratory rate. Improved control can be provided in part by the use of feedback control in the design of the anesthesia delivery system as demonstrated by the development work at the University of Utah.

Feedback control is frequently used in electronic and mechanical design. A certain controlled variable is fed back to the controlling device where it is compared with a reference input.[1,2] The resulting difference or error signal actuates the control elements to change the output so as to reduce the error. Common examples are thermostatically controlled electric frying pans, refrigerators, and household furnaces. Examples in medicine include systems to control anesthesia depth, systolic blood pressure, stimulated muscle action potentials, pulse rate, respiratory rate, and tidal volume. These examples, which include the patient in the feedback loop, have seen moderate success. Systems that do not include the patient in the loop have been more widely accepted, for example, humidifiers, infant warmers, and heated transcutaneous Po_2 monitors. Feedback control functions such that the actuating signal continually adjusts to external conditions. Relatively inexpensive components can be used to obtain better control than is possible by using expensive components in an open loop system.[2]

An analogy can be made between the cruise control on an automobile and the feedback control added to the anesthesia machine. Cruise control maintains the forward velocity of an automobile at some preselected rate. Cruise control does not attempt to replace the driver by observing road conditions or navigating the vehicle, but, rather, it allows the driver to set the velocity of the automobile rather than to adjust the position of the gas pedal. Similarly, the feedback controlled anesthesia machine allows the anesthetist to set the inspired oxygen concentration rather than the oxygen flow, the end-tidal anesthetic gas concentration rather than the vaporizer setting, and the circuit volume rather than the nitrous oxide flow. By allowing the setting of variables that are of greater interest to the anesthetist, the machine becomes simpler to use and is more "user friendly." Feedback control makes the anesthesia machine easier to operate but does not attempt to replace the operator.

This chapter describes the chronologic development of the Utah Anesthesia System and discusses the animal and clinical studies which demonstrate the advantages obtained by using feedback control in the design of an anesthesia machine.

DEVELOPMENT OF THE SYSTEM

Development work on the anesthesia delivery system began in 1974 with research studies concerning the effects of anesthesia on oxygen consumption and the value of oxygen consumption monitoring during high-risk surgery. A block diagram of the instrument is shown in Figure 1.[3] The system used a closed anesthesia breathing circuit (Ohio Cir-

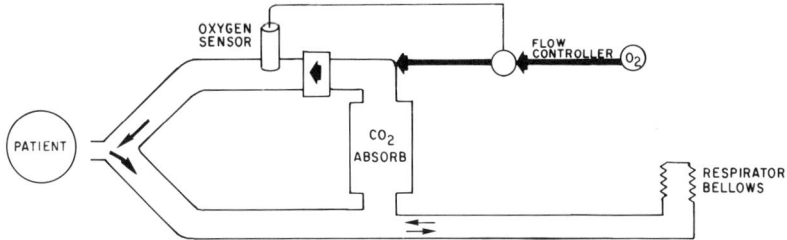

Figure 1. This is a schematic drawing of the closed loop feedback control system for the automatic delivery of oxygen (fresh gas flow) to a closed anesthesia rebreathing system. The oxygen sensor gives a reading of the inspired oxygen concentration, and the feedback control electronics adjusts the oxygen flow through the flow controller until the desired oxygen concentration is achieved. The rate of addition of fresh oxygen is a measure of the patient's oxygen consumption.

cle Absorber, Ohio Medical, Madison, Wisconsin) with the Jumbo carbon dioxide absorber and the standing bellows Air Shields ventilator (Ventimeter Ventilator, Air Shields Inc., Hatboro, Pennsylvania). A Beckman polarographic oxygen sensor (Beckman Instrument, Schiller Park, Illinois) was mounted on the inspiratory limb to measure the oxygen fraction of the inspired air. Feedback control electronics were developed to compare the measured inspired oxygen fraction with the desired oxygen fraction and to provide control of the oxygen flow. A peristaltic roller pump was used to add oxygen to the circuit, the speed of the roller pump being controlled by feedback circuitry. In the steady state, oxygen was added to the closed breathing circuit by the oxygen pump at the rate needed to keep the oxygen concentration constant, and the oxygen flow provided a measure of the patient's oxygen consumption.

The feedback controller, based on a traditional control engineering principle called the "proportional-integral-derivative scheme," produced an output voltage which either sped up or slowed down the pump (Fig. 2).[4] The error signal (e) resulted from measuring the difference between the desired inspired oxygen concentration and the actual measured concentration. The controller then calculated three different aspects of the error signal. A voltage was produced and applied to the output for each of these determinations. The first output voltage was directly proportional to the error signal (e). The second voltage was determined by the rate at which (e) was changing with respect to time (de/dt). The third term took the sum, or integral, of

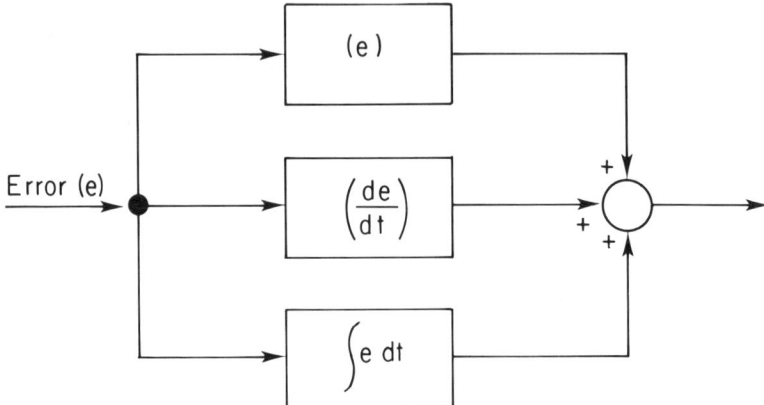

Figure 2. This is a diagram of a proportional-integral-derivative feedback controller. The error signal passes to three feedback control elements. The first element is the proportional term; the second, the derivative term; and the third, the integral term. The sum of these three elements forms the output of the feedback controller.

the error accumulated over time, $\int e\,dt$, and supplied a voltage proportional to this accumulated error.

Appropriate constants K_1, K_2, and K_3 were determined empirically for balancing the three different aspects of the error signal, using root-locus techniques and bode plots. The resultant control signal (output) was applied to the pump to control oxygen inflow to the circuit.

This system for measuring the patient's oxygen consumption was shown in a patient validation study to have an accuracy greater than ± 6 percent.[5] In addition, the system was used as a tool to study the effect of endotoxic shock on oxygen consumption in Rhesus monkeys,[6] the effect of thiopental and fentanyl boluses on oxygen consumption in dogs,[7] the effect of dopamine, atropine, and phenylephrine and cardiac pacing on oxygen consumption during fentanyl-nitrous oxide anesthesia in the dog,[8] and the effect of deep hypothermia and microwave rewarming on oxygen consumption.[9] It was used in patients to study the change in oxygen consumption following bolus intravenous infusions of sodium thiopental and fentanyl during oxygen-narcotic anesthesia.[10] Response to step changes in oxygen consumption occurred within 20 seconds, but 4.5 minutes were required to reach 95 percent of the new $\dot{V}O_2$ value. Continuous monitoring of oxygen consumption appeared to be a useful indicator of depth of anesthesia and warned of low cardiac output, hypoxia, and decreased oxygen transport.

The system was expanded in 1975 when a second feedback loop was added for the delivery of nitrous oxide (Fig. 3).[11] This feedback loop consisted of a volume sensor, a feedback control circuit, and a nitrous oxide pump. The breathing circuit volume was sensed by a linear array of 10 photosensitive duodiodes placed on the opposite side of the respirator bellows from a fluorescent lantern. The feedback circuit compared a voltage proportional with the actual circuit volume and used this difference through a proportional-integral-derivative controller to adjust the speed of a peristaltic roller pump. The revolutions per minute of this constant stroke volume pump were measured by a tachometer and displayed in milliliters of nitrous oxide per minute.

Responses to changes in circuit volume were rapid and immediate.[12] It was important that the closed-circuit volume be maintained so that ventilation could continue. With the occurrence of a patient disconnection and reconnection, the circuit completely and automatically refilled with the desired oxygen concentration within 30 seconds.

Through use of the prototype system we found the peristaltic roller pumps to be a weak component in the system. As the tubing and the pump tended to wear, the calibration of the pump changed and the revolutions per minute no longer represented an accurate measure of the fresh gas flow. In 1978, thermal mass flow control units (Brooks Instrument, Hatfield, Pennsylvania) were used to replace the roller pumps. The flow controllers used a solenoid actuated variable orifice in line with a thermal flow sensor. The position of the needle valve was

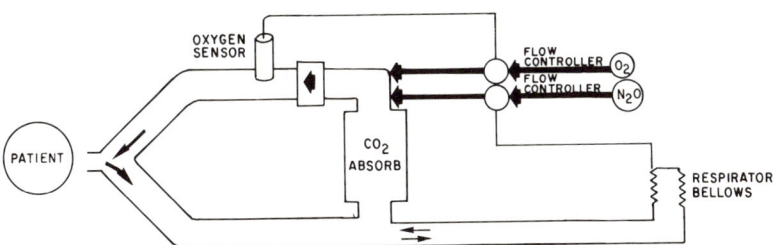

Figure 3. This is a schematic drawing of a closed-circuit anesthesia breathing system showing feedback control of oxygen and nitrous oxide fresh gas flows. The nitrous oxide feedback control loop measures the circuit volume from a transducer on the respirator bellows and adjusts the nitrous oxide fresh gas flow to achieve a constant circuit volume.

adjusted by feedback control to achieve the desired flow rate. Each unit was calibrated over a 0 to 1000 ml per minute flow range and had an accuracy of ± 1 percent of full scale. Gases were supplied to these units from a source at 50 psi. A rotameter was placed on the instrument's front panel to provide a visual indication of gas flow from both the oxygen and the nitrous oxide flow controllers. These newer flow controllers gave a much more accurate measure of fresh gas flows and enhanced oxygen consumption and nitrous oxide uptake monitoring.

This system was used to deliver oxygen-xenon anesthesia.[13] Xenon was used in place of nitrous oxide (see Figure 2). Because of the cost of xenon ($12 per liter), the closed-circuit system and electronic control made it feasible to study xenon anesthesia.

A third feedback loop was implemented in 1978 to control mechanical ventilation (Fig. 4).[14,15] The feedback system used an 8085 microprocessor to control the inspired minute volume of a Siemens

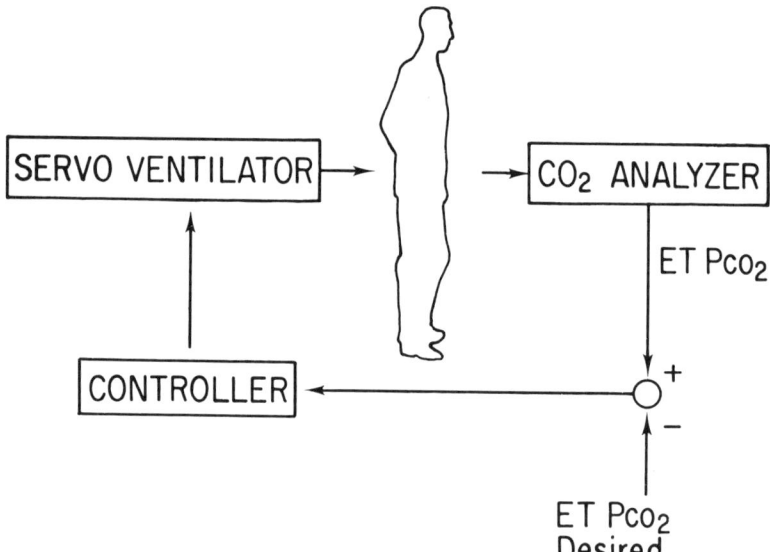

Figure 4. This is a diagram of a closed feedback loop for the control of mechanical ventilation. A patient's end-tidal pCO_2 ($ETPCO_2$) is measured by a carbon dioxide analyzer and compared with the desired $ETPCO_2$. This different signal goes to a proportional-integral-derivative controller which adjusts the patient ventilator. This closed loop system achieves and maintains a constant $ETPCO_2$.

900B Servoventilator (Siemens-Elema, Solna, Sweden). End-tidal carbon dioxide ($ETCO_2$) was measured at the airway by an infrared Siemens 930 carbon dioxide analyzer. Measured $ETCO_2$ was compared with the desired $ETCO_2$ to produce an error signal. A proportional-integral-derivative controller produced a signal to adjust the timing cycle of the Servoventilator. The inspired minute volume was reset every 5 seconds.

The controller was evaluated in a dog study in which it was found that closed loop control of ventilation based on $ETCO_2$ measurements successfully compensated for increases in carbon dioxide production, keeping the arterial Pco_2 constant.[16] The controller did not, however, keep $Paco_2$ at the desired level when significant changes occurred in the distribution of blood flow to ventilation (V/Q). It was anticipated that additional inputs to the controller such as carbon dioxide excretion and oxygen consumption would improve the controller's performance and make it more applicable for routine clinical use.

In 1980, a fourth control loop was added to the system to control anesthetic vapor concentration (Fig. 5). Vapor concentration in the anesthesia circuit was measured by a prototype gas analyzer (Siemens Corporation, Solna, Sweden) which used a dispersive infrared absorption technique. The gas analysis head was placed in the anesthesia circuit inspiratory limb next to the carbon dioxide absorber. The

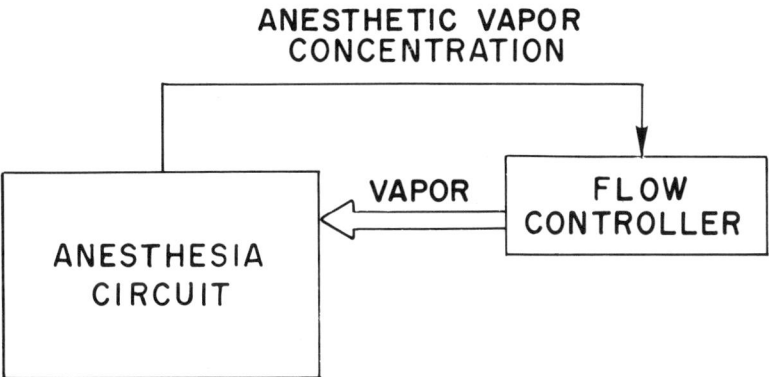

Figure 5. This is a blocked diagram of the feedback control scheme used to adjust anesthetic vapor concentration. The inspired or end-tidal anesthetic vapor concentration is measured by an infrared detector. The flow rate of oxygen through a copper kettle vaporizer is adjusted to achieve and to maintain the desired anesthetic vapor concentration in the closed anesthesia circuit.

feedback controller varied the oxygen flow of a dual mass flow controller (0 to 100 ml per minute and 0 to 1000 ml per minute ranges). The oxygen flow passed through a copper kettle vaporizer to the expiratory limb of the circuit and thus maintained the desired inspiratory circuit vapor concentration. The flow rate of volatile anesthetic agent to the circuit was calculated from the oxygen flow rate, the copper kettle temperature, and the anesthetic vapor partial pressure. The oxygen flow rate through the copper kettle was plotted continuously so that the anesthetist had a continuous display of the anesthetic uptake curve. The shape of the uptake curve and its slope at any point in time gave the anesthesiologist equilibration information for managing cardiovascular depression and balancing against surgical stimulation.

In a follow-up study, the infrared gas analyzer was placed between the patient and the circuit Y piece.[17,18] A peak detector circuit was used to obtain a continuous measure of end-tidal vapor concentration. Feedback control was used to adjust automatically the inspired vapor concentration to achieve and to maintain the desired end-tidal vapor concentration. This system delivered anesthesia using an automated "overpressure" technique. In a series of 14 dogs, we compared anesthesia induction using a constant inspired vapor concentration versus a constant end-tidal concentration. The two methods of anesthesia control did not produce statistically significant differences in heart rate, blood pressure, or cardiac output. The "overpressure" technique used in this study, whereby the end-tidal concentration was controlled by feedback techniques, produced a rapid induction of anesthesia without cardiovascular depression. The use of feedback control to automatically adjust the end-tidal enflurane concentration has since been used quite extensively in patients. By clinical experience, it appears to be a safe technique for anesthesia induction.

CURRENT SYSTEM CONFIGURATION

A conceptual diagram of the current Utah Anesthesia System is shown in Figure 6. Three feedback loops are used to adjust the fresh gas flows to a closed anesthesia breathing circuit. Initially the user sets the desired inspired oxygen concentration and the desired inspired or end-tidal vapor concentration. The fresh gas flow of oxygen to the circuit is adjusted by feedback control to maintain the desired inspired oxygen concentration. The volume of the closed circuit is maintained by feedback control of the nitrous oxide–fresh gas flow. The inhala-

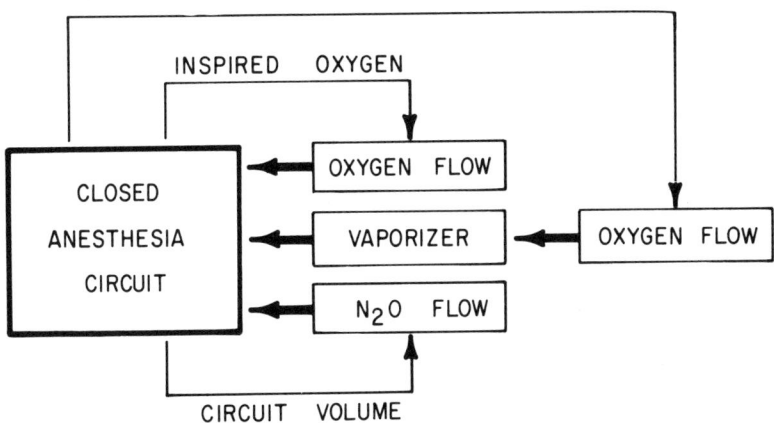

Figure 6. This is a conceptual blocked diagram of the three feedback control loops which operate simultaneously to adjust the fresh gas flow to a closed anesthesia circuit.

tion agent concentration is measured in either the inspired gas or end-tidal gas, and the flow of oxygen through a copper kettle vaporizer is adjusted to achieve the desired vapor concentrations. Electronic control is used to adjust the fresh gas flows and to maintain the circuit volume, inspired oxygen concentration, and end-tidal or inspired inhalation agent concentrations. The control of ventilation is provided by a fourth feedback loop. Because of the interdependence of anesthetic uptake and alveolar ventilation, it seems desirable in the future to examine the interaction between the four control loops. This system also monitors the patient's oxygen consumption, nitrous oxide uptake, and inhalation agent uptake. It appears that anesthesia is delivered more accurately, economically, and safely because of the automation and closed loop control which has been added to the anesthesia machine.

CLINICAL APPLICATION

Through the clinical use of this system we have accumulated considerable data concerning oxygen consumption, nitrous oxide uptake, and anesthesia uptake during surgery. Oxygen consumption generally will increase with light anesthesia and will decrease with increased anesthetic depth[7,10] or depression of oxygen transport.[6] During balanced anesthesia with thiopental or fentanyl, one generally finds an 8 percent to 10 percent decrease in oxygen consumption following intravenous boluses of the agents.[10] During light anesthesia a pain stimulus generally will increase oxygen consumption, but pain will have little effect during deep anesthesia.[7] Decreases with hypothermia and septic shock have also been documented.[6,9]

The nitrous oxide uptake curve has not been used except for detecting leaks in the circuit. If the nitrous oxide uptake is exceptionally high, it is a strong indication that leaks exist in the closed anesthesia circuit.[12]

The uptake curve for the inhalation agent gives an indication of the individual patient's anesthetic condition. The observation that the rapid uptake phase is complete gives one confidence that the patient has reached equilibrium with the selected anesthesia concentration. Surgery should be delayed until after the rapid uptake phase has been completed and the induction is more nearly stable.

The Utah system has shown the feasibility of adding feedback control to the anesthesia machine. Closed loop control of the breathing circuit oxygen concentration, volume, and volatile agent concentration have provided functions for the anesthesia machine which make it easier to use. The fresh gas flows are adjusted automatically without user intervention. This function is particularly useful when using closed-circuit anesthesia because fresh gas flow rates are automatically matched to the patient's metabolic gas exchange and uptake. Extensive clinical experience has shown the system to be safe and adequately responsive over a range of patients from children to adults.

Closed loop control provided an "overpressure" technique for delivering the volatile agent by controlling end-tidal gas concentrations. The inspired gas concentration, which is feedback controlled, is initially at a much higher level than the desired arterial concentration to provide a rapid induction. It appears that induction time is reduced without undue hazard to the patient.

In addition to better control, the system adds monitoring capability to the anesthesia machine. Trends in oxygen consumption, nitrous oxide uptake, and anesthetic agent uptake better define the patient's physiologic condition under anesthesia.

THE FUTURE

An ideal anesthesia machine would have provision for the user to set a desired level of anesthesia while ensuring adequate oxygen delivery to the tissue and maintenance of carbon dioxide homeostasis. (Other aspects of anesthesia, for example, neuromuscular blockade, blood volume, and body temperature, are not considered because they are not generally provided through the airway.) A monitor of anesthetic depth is needed before the first goal can be met. The energy spectrum of the electroencephalogram has been investigated but to date has proved unsatisfactory.[19] Perhaps new approaches to processing this signal will produce better results. If we cannot measure the physiologic response to anesthesia, the next best approach is to measure brain or arterial blood concentrations. Transcutaneous electrodes can possibly be developed to make the measurement noninvasively. The simplest solution using present technology is to use end-tidal anesthetic monitoring.

Adequate oxygen delivery to the tissues is influenced strongly by the inspired oxygen concentration, oxygen diffusion, shunt, and cardiac output. Delivery of a high inspired oxygen concentration alone does not ensure adequate delivery to tissues. Direct Pa_{O_2} measurements leave only cardiac output and peripheral shunt in question. The ear oximeter and transcutaneous electrodes are noninvasive means for obtaining Pa_{O_2} and can be reliable under proper conditions. The set-up time for transcutaneous monitors is an undesirable factor at present. Because of the complexity of this monitoring, it may be quite some time before routine monitoring will include more than inspired oxygen concentration. Monitoring $\dot{V}_{O_2}$ may help in this sector because it reflects both oxygen consumption and transport.

Carbon dioxide homeostasis can generally be achieved with end-tidal P_{CO_2} monitoring and mechanical control of ventilation. Transcutaneous P_{CO_2} or intra-arterial P_{CO_2} are more direct measurements. Transcutaneous P_{CO_2} does not give an absolute value, though it is a better trend monitor than end-tidal,[20] and intra-arterial monitoring is, of course, invasive. End-tidal carbon dioxide would seem to be the preferred monitor of carbon dioxide homeostasis when care is used to ensure the absence of increased dead space, high respiratory rates, large V/Q abnormalities, and other complicating factors. The shape of the excretory carbon dioxide curve and $\dot{V}_{CO_2}$ may be helpful in correcting $ETCO_2$ inaccuracies.

CONCLUSION

The Utah system is only the first step in approaching these goals of an ideal anesthesia machine. The Utah system has shown the feasibility of adding feedback control to the anesthesia machine to adjust variables which are of greater significance to the anesthetist than fresh gas flows. As monitoring technology improves and anesthesia machines are upgraded accordingly, these machines should become much easier to use, and, we hope, anesthetic safety thus will be improved.

REFERENCES

1. EVELEIGH, VW: *Introduction to control systems design.* McGraw-Hill, New York, 1972, pp 1–9.
2. RAVEN, FH: *Automatic control engineering.* McGraw-Hill, New York, 1961, pp 1–5.
3. WESTENSKOW, DR, ET AL: *Instrumentation for continuous monitoring of oxygen consumption.* IEEE 1975 Region Six (Western USA) Conference 25, 1975.
4. GEHMLICH, DK AND HAMMON, SB: *Electromechanical systems.* McGraw-Hill, New York, 1967, pp 91–100.
5. WESTENSKOW, DR, ET AL: *Instrumentation for measuring continuous oxygen consumption of surgical patients.* IEEE Transaction, Biomedical Engineering (24)4:331–337, 1977.
6. WESTENSKOW, DR, ET AL: *Dynamic metabolic response to septic shock in the primate.* 30th Annual Conference on Engineering in Medicine and Biology 19:200, 1977.
7. WESTENSKOW, DR, ET AL: *Correlation of oxygen uptake and cardiovascular dynamics during N_2O-fentanyl and N_2O-thiopental anesthesia in the dog.* Anesth Analg 57(1):37–41, 1978.
8. WESTENSKOW, DR, HUFFAKER, JK, STANLEY, TH: *The effect of dopamine, atropine, phenylephrine and cardiac pacing on oxygen consumption during fentanyl-nitrous oxide anesthesia in the dog.* Can Anaesth Soc J 28(2):121–124, 1981.
9. WESTENSKOW, DR, *Physiologic effects of deep hypothermia and microwave rewarming: Possible application for neonatal cardiac surgery.* Anesth Analg 58(4):297–301, 1979.
10. WESTENSKOW, DR AND JORDAN, WS: *Changes in oxygen consumption induced by fentanyl and thiopentone during balanced anaesthesia.* Can Anaesth Soc J 25(1):18–21, 1978.
11. WESTENSKOW, DR, ET AL: *Whole body oxygen consumption during anesthesia.* 29th Annual Conference on Engineering in Medicine and Biology 18:158, 1976.
12. WESTENSKOW, DR, JORDAN, WS, GEHMLICH, DS: *Electronic feedback control and measurement of oxygen consumption during closed circuit*

anesthesia. In ALDRETE, JA, LOWE, HJ, VIRTUE, RW: Low Flow and Closed Circuit Anesthesia. Grune & Stratton, New York, pp 135–146, 1979.

13. WESTENSKOW, DR, ET AL: *Xenon rebreathing system for liver blood flow measurement.* 32nd Annual Conference on Engineering in Medicine and Biology 21:100, 1979.
14. WESTENSKOW, DR, ET AL: *Closed loop therapy in the critical care unit using microprocessor controllers,* Ed by NAIR, S. Plenum Pub, New York, 1980, pp 79–87.
15. WESTENSKOW, DR, ET AL: *Microprocessors in intensive care medicine.* Med Instrum 14(6):311–313, 1980.
16. OHLSON, KB, WESTENSKOW, DR, JORDAN, WS: *Feedback control of ventilation using expired CO_2l.* Anaesthesiology (Suppl) 53(3S):S387, 1980.
17. WESTENSKOW, DR, JORDAN, WS, HAYES, JK: *Closed loop control of the closed circuit anesthesia breathing circuit.* Proceedings 17th Annual Meeting of Association Medical Instrumentation, May, 1982.
18. WESTENSKOW, DR, HAYES, JK, JORDAN, WS: *Inspired vs end-tidal control of enflurane anesthesia in dogs.* Anesth Analg (in press).
19. CHILCOAT, RT: *Servo loops in the control of anaesthetic parameters.* Thesis, Department of Anesthesiology, State University of NY, Upstate Medical Center, Syracuse, NY.
20. WESTENSKOW, DR, JORDAN, WS, PACE, NL: *Intraoperative monitoring of arterial P_{CO_2}: Comparing end-tidal and transcutaneous sensors.* Anesth Analg 61(2):223, 1982.

SECTION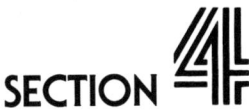

THE FUTURE LIES AHEAD

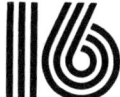

WHAT DO WE DO UNTIL THE FUTURE GETS HERE?
Reynolds J. Saunders, M.D.

PLANNING FOR THE FUTURE

Although there are encouraging prospects for new developments in anesthesia delivery systems, the clinician still is forced to deal with a series of urgent questions. Confronted with the realization that all is not as it should be, each anesthesiologist must deal with several problems in planning for the future. The basic question, as always in life, is "What do I do next?"

Problems with planning include uncertainty about the future rate and direction of progress; the rapidity with which progress already is occurring; obsolescence of systems with high initial cost and a traditionally long lifetime; and re-education and retraining of clinicians in use of new technology. The uncertainties involved are no more distressing than in other fields enduring rapid technologic advancement. Although mistakes in equipment selection undoubtedly will be made, alertness in their detection should reduce adverse impact on patient care. In any case, one must balance the effects of errors in selection of systems ("Gee, if I'd only waited six more months!" or "If I had known this 'frammis' was going to be such a useless attachment, I would never have spent the money!") against the effect of retaining a system with known hazards.[1]

DO YOU NEED TO CHANGE?

Before rushing out to buy the newest Whizmatron anesthesia machine after perusing a full-color brochure that outweighs the machine, the clinician must consider whether existing equipment might serve for a bit longer. This heretical question should be answered by a dispassionate evaluation: first, one's clinical requirements and safety considerations, followed by frequency-of-repair record and cost of maintenance. Machines not meeting standards set by the Joint Commission on the Accreditation of Hospitals (JCAH) are in gross violation of safety standards; machines not meeting Z79 standards should make the anesthesiologist anxious. Although perusal of earlier chapters in this volume may trigger profound dissatisfaction with the status quo, existing equipment may be reasonably safe; it may be recently purchased; it may have met one's needs until now, when perceived needs have expanded to meet new knowledge. The best course here is to sit back, to acquire no new equipment, and to perform a detailed inventory of need while satisfactory equipment is further amortized.

DEALING WITH EQUIPMENT PROBLEMS

It is important, both for improved anesthesia care and for fiscal planning, that vague feelings of dissatisfaction be translated into specific defects requiring remedies. Rendell-Baker[1] provides a detailed review of problems with anesthesia machines from a design standpoint and offers an overview[2,3] of standards, proposed and enacted, for anesthesia equipment. Armed with this information, a systematic review can be made of the clinician's existing equipment. New features can then be assigned to one of the following four categories:

1. safety
2. obsolescence
3. convenience
4. glamor.

New features can be either those hoped for or those offered by a manufacturer; in either case, they should be classified as above.

Safety

Responsible clinicians always are concerned about safety in a notoriously hazardous occupation. In evaluating anesthesia delivery systems, one must ask two basic questions:

1. Is my system unsafe because of imprecision, inaccuracy or unreliability?
2. Is my system unsafe because of deficiencies in controllability, surveillance, or information about machine function?

While the first category is more often considered in case reports of disaster and in our routine morning check of equipment, the second category is worth careful consideration. Human operators, because they have inconstant vigilance and limited capacity to absorb and to use information, may make serious mistakes as a result of confusing information display, ambiguous or imprecise controls, or lack of vigilance aids.

Obsolescence

True obsolescence exists when

1. improved function is needed;
2. a new function is available;
3. the new function is an improvement.

Often our notion that our machinery is obsolete fails one or more of these tests, in which case obsolescence should not be a factor in selection of new devices. If, however, a machine or system truly is obsolete, the clinician should exert all effort possible to replace it with a modern device.

In association with the word "planned," obsolescence conveys the image of greedy, conniving manufacturers contriving to milk the consumer's checkbook. Careful examination of the high-unit-cost, low-sales-volume anesthesia industry reveals not planned obsolescence but poorly planned progress, with manufacturers uncertain about goals and lagging behind the progress of technology in other industries. After decades of minimal progress and stasis in design we suddenly are deluged with "new" anesthesia systems, which are basically the same old systems with cosmetic overlays. Although some safety features gradually are tacked on to the old designs, they often reveal severe gaps between the design engineers' perception of need and the realities of the operating suite. Often new features do not perform as represented, attempt to fill a nonexistent need, or are difficult to use effectively.

Convenience

Inconvenience can wreak havoc with the most carefully laid plans when a complex series of actions must be undertaken. The distraction caused by constantly having to fuss and to fiddle with equipment, to spend valuable time setting up and calibrating, or to confirm proper function frequently can be detrimental both to the morale of the anesthetist and to the health of the patient. A vigilant and intellectually active anesthetist will be freed by convenience features to attend to patients rather than to machines; the slothful anesthetist may be stimulated by vigilance alarms, the automatic features of which may diminish occurrence of disasters. It is no sin to relish convenience when it enhances patient care, case turnover time, or information gathering. Gas monitors, calculators, automatic gas concentration control, anesthesia record generation, and other convenience features are not to be spurned just because the anesthetist's job is made easier.

Glamor

Many medical centers take pride in having the newest and best equipment, and they attract clinical staff and patients partly on this basis. Without condoning this "medical arms race," it must be recognized that this factor exists in other areas of the hospital.[4] Unfortunately, much of the sales approach of anesthesia equipment manufacturers recently has used glamor as a selling point. It is worthwhile to consult with hospital biomedical engineers who are familiar with anesthesia equipment (not all are) and to try to discern the feathers from the bird.

DEVELOPING SPECIFICATIONS

It is well to develop a clear set of operational specifications prior to purchase for modification of anesthetic equipment. From these specifications it should become clear where deficiencies lie in current equipment. A determination then can be made whether modification is possible or whether a new system must be acquired. Guides to selection should be consulted[5,4] so that as little as possible is overlooked. The American National Standards Institute Z79 standards should be acquired (see Chapter 4) and studied, as should the standards of the Joint Commission on Accreditation of Hospitals. Finally, an in-depth survey should be made of user preferences, work habits, and perceived needs of anesthetists at the hospital. Standardization is helpful in accident prevention but rarely possible fiscally, owing to the inability to replace simultaneously all the gas machines in the operating suite. It must be remembered however, that JCAH standards specify that the same quality of equipment shall be available in all anesthetizing locations within the hospital. The potential for conflicting goals here is obvious but must be faced squarely.

There are several attributes for which we should ask when buying a delivery system. These should help decrease trauma in the future as new developments appear. Foremost among desirable characteristics is *modularity,* the ability to interchange or exchange components of the system without adversely affecting the rest of the system. Modularity facilitates repair and updating of equipment without major upheaval. A few monitoring systems and certain calibrated vaporizers have this capability, which also may allow physical placement of components to suit the anesthesiologist's preference.

Communication is another key feature. Does each component of the system (monitor, gas delivery, sensors, ventilator) have an interface which allows communication with other devices and with a computer? Standard interfaces include RS232, IEEE-488, HPIB, HPIL, and other modes of communication used for years in the electronics industry to facilitate communication between electronic devices.

Electronic control is a feature often maligned because of poorly designed "idiot lights" in autos, useless controls on microwave ovens, and other monuments to poor engineering. Yet properly designed electronic systems usually last longer between repairs than equivalent mechanical systems.

Redundancy of systems allows one component to check the performance of its twin, allows continued operation in case of component failure, and provides a measure of security.

HOW TO DIG THROUGH MANUFACTURERS' HYPERBOLE

Although manufacturers of anesthesia delivery systems are concerned about efficacy and safety of their devices, it must be recognized that altruism competes for their attention with the bottom line on the stockholders' report. They can hardly be expected to herald introduction of a new device with a frank confession of its deficits. Neither will they remind you that, with the low sales volume and high retooling costs, innovation cuts profit margins. We must be perspicacious in reading their literature and talking to their sales representatives, who are not anesthetizing our patients and who hold their company's best interests above those of us or our patients.

The key word in dealing with manufacturers is *data*. We must strike out for truth in advertising by carefully inspecting claims and demanding to see the evidence supporting them. Drug manufacturers are required to provide results of prospective, double-blind, crossover, placebo-controlled clinical trials to support claims of efficacy and safety. We should demand an equivalent depth of information regarding anesthesia delivery systems. For instance, if a manufacturer claims that the machine provides accurate gas flows, we should ask

1. How accurate?
2. By what standard were they measured?
3. Are machines on the assembly line subjected to the same testing?
4. What are the results of this production testing?
5. Will my machine have its accuracy results shipped with it?
6. How long can I expect the machine to stay within these limits of accuracy?
7. What data supports that time estimate?
8. Will the company guarantee the accuracy?
9. How will I know when the machine becomes inaccurate? (Does it self-check with a redundant system?)

If they claim that human factors engineering was used in system development, we should ask for data showing how human performance was affected by this new design, as opposed to others. The questions above should provide an example of the sort of detail the clinician should expect from the manufacturer, but many sales representatives become confused, hostile, or hurt that we would question their company's integrity.

WHAT TO DO WHEN A SYSTEM IS SELECTED

In the past, anesthesia machines (and many other equipment items) could be kept until they wore out, with certainty that few improvements would have occurred during the life of the device. We are likely to see over the next eight to ten years (the usual lifetime for an anesthesia machine, although a few are maintained up to twenty years) the same rate of progress that we are seeing in physiologic monitors and ventilators. In those fields, we find that rapid technologic progress renders current equipment truly obsolete before it can wear out. Increasing use of solid-state components has increased the functional lifetime of devices because there are fewer mechanical parts to fail.

A radical change in philosophy of ownership may be required to avoid being trapped with expensive, obsolete anesthesia equipment. The burden of depreciation and amortization might properly be shifted to the equipment supplier or leasing company. Benefits from leasing arrangements include frequent updating of equipment; avoidance of large, irregularly cyclic capital equipment burdens; and the ability to budget equipment costs on a consistent basis. Until the goal is realized of modular systems with replaceable or reprogrammable components, anesthesia delivery systems will require replacement to update them. This replacement might better be accomplished upon expiration of fixed- or variable-term leases, which shift the burden of obsolescence away from the anesthesiologist or hospital. Most leasing agreements, however, equate with purchase price at about 24 months. The tax advantages of investment tax credits, accelerated depreciation, and interest charges on purchased equipment must be balanced against the resistance of hospital equipment committees to junking functional but obsolete equipment. Creative financing alternatives for keeping abreast of current technology should be explored.

SUMMARY

We have seen that there are serious design inadequacies in the basic anesthesia machines now in the marketplace. None of these meets criteria for technologic soundness or clinical utility elaborated in previous chapters. It is tempting to simply buy what is available and shrug one's shoulders over the situation. Those in desperate need of replacement equipment should go ahead and buy, because significant changes may be years away. However, those who are able and disposed to wait for real progress may accelerate the process by waiting not silently but loudly.

Until the anesthesiologists on the firing line are consistently asking technically sophisticated questions related to safety and efficacy, expecting them to be answered, and letting their equipment budgets speak where words do not, we can expect consistent *laissez-faire* attitudes and actions from the anesthesia machine industry. Technology already available in other industries will continue to be overlooked or ignored, and our clinical needs will be unmet until industry is convinced that the majority of anesthetists want far-reaching substantive change in anesthesia delivery system design. We have no choice but to use what is currently available; but we can reward solid, thoughtful innovation with our capital equipment dollars, with our support of research in anesthesia technology, with our verbal and written requests to manufacturers, and with our individual time spent staying abreast of technologic issues. The ultimate beneficiaries are our patients; we cannot remain static—we must improve.

REFERENCES

1. RENDELL-BAKER, L: *Problems with anesthetic gas machines and their solutions.* Int Anesthesiol Clin 20(3):1–82, 1982.
2. RENDELL-BAKER, L. *Standards for Anesthesia: The Issues.* Chapter 4 of this volume.
3. RENDELL-BAKER, L: *Standards for anesthetic and ventilatory equipment.* Int Anesthesiol Clin 20(3):171–204, 1982.
4. BAUMAN, R: *How to choose the best equipment for the operating room and critical care unit.* In OSNOWITZ, D (ED): *Medical Products Reference, Anesthesiology and Critical Care.* Warren Gorhan & Lamont, Boston, 1982.
5. SATWICZ, PR AND SHAGRIN, JM: *The selection of anesthetic equipment.* Int Anesthesiol Clin 19(2):97–112, 1981.

INDEX

Italics indicate a figure. A t indicates a table.

ABORTION, spontaneous, waste gases and, 112
Absorption system, adult circle, 64
Acetone, rebreathing systems and, 25
Advertising, hyperbole and, 241–242
Agents. *See also* specific agents.
 concentration of, computers and, 55
 halogenated
  greenhouse effect and, 117–118
  ozone destruction and, 118
 neuromuscular blocking, computers and, 55
 mass flow rates of, 142, 146–148
 volatile. *See* Volatile agent.
Air Shields Ventimeter ventilator, 223
Airway pressure, monitoring of, computers and, 54
Alabama Automated Closed-Circuit Anesthesia System
 bellows position sensor and, 180
 components of, 179–181, *180*
 computer control in, 181–182
 diagram of, *180*
 oxygen monitoring in, 180–182, *182*
 standard anesthesia machine and, 179
 ventilation and, 181
 volatile agent analyzer and, 181

Alarms
 Boston system and, 213, 217–218
 disconnection, 70
 oxygen analyzer, 69
 pulmonary barotrauma, 70–71
 Utah system and, 223–224
Anesthesia machine. *See also* specific systems.
 ventilator and
  accessory nature of, 170–171
  integration of, 171–172
Arizona system
 basis of, theoretical, 185–186
 components of, 198–204, *199, 200, 203*. *See also* individual components.
 computer and, 204–205
 gas proportionating system of
  components of, 200–201, *200*
  criteria for, 198–200, *200*
 history of, 185
 human interaction in, 186–187
 microprocessor and, 204–205
 sensors of
  blood pressure and, 196, *197*
  central nervous system and, 196–198
  electrocardiographic, 195–196

245

Arizona system—*continued*
  endotracheal multiprobes and, 195–196
  esophageal multiprobes and, 195–196
  evaluation of, 187
  flow, 194–195
  gas
    electromechanical, 191–194, *193*
    flueric oscillator, 188–191, *189, 190*
    linear resistor-orifice, 191, *192*
  ion specific field effect transistors and, 195
  physiologic, 195–198, *197*
  ventilators in
    design guidelines for, 202, 202t
    high-frequency, 203–204
    pediatric, 203, *203*
  volatile agents in
    delivery of, 201
    recovery of, 201–202
Association for the Advancement of Medical Instrumentation, engineering standards and, 69
Ayre's T-piece, 12, *13,* 14

BAIN system, 12, *13*
Balanced anesthesia, rebreathing system and, 28, 28t
Barotrauma, pulmonary, alarm for, 70–71, 70t
Birth defects, waste gases and, 112
Blood gas, measurement of, computers and, 54. *See also* specific blood gases.
Blood pressure, monitoring of
  Arizona system and, 196
  automatic, 69
Bohr equation, ventilation status and, 144
Boston system
  alarms and, 213, 217–218
  breathing circuit of, 213–214
  display and, 214–216, *216*
  flexibility of, 213
  flow rates in, 211
  future of, 218
  guidelines for, 207–209, *208*
  microprocessor control of, 211–213
  modes in, 214
  prototype of
    design of, 209–211, *210, 215, 216*
    function of, 214–218, *216*
  safety and, 213
  volatile agents in
    delivery of, 211–212
    differentiation of, 212
Bounding bobbin, flowmeters and, 102–103
Breathing circuit. *See also* Rebreathing systems.
  design of, 94
  disconnections of, accidental, 68
  layout standards for, 65–67
  performance standards of, 67–68

CARBON dioxide
  absorption of
    closed-circuit system and, 12, *13,* 119
    recycling gas and, 119
    Utah system and, 223
  concentration of
    analyzer for, 181
    computers and, 54
    depth of anesthesia and, 140, 141t
    monitoring of, 138, 139t, 140, 170
    ventilation rate and, 178–179
  mass flow rates of, 142
  measurement of, *20,* 21
  rebreathing systems and, 25
  Utah system and, 231
  ventilators and, design of, 96–97
Cardiovascular system, monitoring of, computers and, 55–56. *See also* Electrocardiograph.
Central nervous system, monitoring of, Arizona system and, 196–198
Charcoal shunt, rebreathing systems and, 26–28, *26, 27,* 31
Classification of delivery systems, 11–12, 12t
Closed-circuit system. *See* Rebreathing system.
Coanda effect, flueric oscillator and, 188
Cognitive tunnel vision, 161
Communication, equipment design and, 241

Compressed Gas Association, breathing system fittings and, 66
Compressed spectral array, 197-198
Computers. *See also* Control systems; Data processing; specific systems.
  acid-base balance and, 56
  agent concentration in, 55
  airway pressure in, 54
  Alabama system and, 177-182
  algorithms and, 53, 57
  analog, definition of, 42-44, *43*
  analog-digital converters in, *43,* 44
  binary system in, 44-45, *45*
  bits and, 44-47, *45, 46*
  blood gas measurements in, 54
  body temperature and, 56
  Boston system and, 212-213
  bytes and, 45-47, *46*
  capabilities of, general, 52
  cardiovascular system and, 55-56
  cognitive tunnel vision and, 161
  control systems and, 56-57, 95-96, 128-129
  data collection in, 53-54
  data recording and, 53-54
  decimal system in, 44-45, *45*
  decision making and, 150-151
  design of future, 95-96
  digital, definition of, 42-44, *43*
  display and, 152, 160-161
  electroencephalograms and, 196-197
  electrolyte levels and, 56
  function of, general, 40-42, *40,* 152-153
  funnel function of, 152-153
  history of, 39-40
  human engineering and
    display and, 160-161
    problems of, 159
    record keeping and, 161
  instructions for, 49-50
  limitations of, general, 52-53
  microprocessor control and, design of, 95-96
  muscle relaxation in, 55
  need for, anesthesia and, 57
  nybbles in, 45
  oxygen delivery and, 54, 179
  prediction and, 150-151
  programming of
    BASIC in, 52
    bootstrap loader in, 50, *51*
    bugs in, 52
    central processing unit and, 47-50, *48*
    COBOL in, 52
    compiler in, 52
    error message in, 52
    files in, 50-52
    FORTRAN in, 52
    "garbage in, garbage out (GIGO)" in, 52-53
    object code in, 52
    operating system in, 50, *51*
    source code in, 52
  record keeping and, 161
  structure of
    accumulator in, 49
    cathode ray tube in, 42
    central processing unit in, 47-50, *48*
    converters in, *43,* 44
    diagram of, *41*
    input/output devices in, *41,* 42-44, *43*
    instructions and, 49-50
    magnetic disk drives in, 42
    magnetic tape drives in, 42
    memory in, 44-47, *45, 46*
    plotters in, 42
    printers in, 42
    program counter in, 49
    punched card readers in, 42
    storage area in, 44-47, *45, 46*
  urine output and, 56
  variables and, availability of, 151-152
  ventilation and, 54, 179
  volatile agent delivery and, 179
Concentration
  agent, monitoring of, 24, 28-31, 29t, 30t. *See also* specific agents.
  gas. *See* specific gases.
  minimal alveolar, 29t, 30, 30t, 194. *See also* specific agents.
Conservation of mass
  gas flow and, 141, 146
  principle of, 100-101
Control systems
  benefits of, 133-134
  closed loop
    definition of, *127,* 128
    feedback in, 128
    oxygen concentration in, 131
    time delays in, 128

Control systems—*continued*
  computers and, 56–57, 95–96, 128–129
  cost-benefit ratio of, 134
  current, anesthesia and, 130–133, *132*
  definition of, 127–129
  end-tidal anesthetic concentration in, 132
  future, anesthesia and, 134
  history of, 125
  microprocessors and, 128–129
  neuromuscular block and, 134
  open loop, definition of, 127–128, *127*
  physiologic factors and, 126, 129–132
  types of, 127, *127*
Convenience features, equipment selection and, 240
Cost effectiveness, delivery systems and, 5–6

DALTON'S law, partial pressure and, 147
Data, availability of, human response to, 151–152
Data processing. *See also* Computers.
  electrocardiogram and, 154–155, *154*
  modeling in, 156–159, *157, 158*
  need for, 153–154
  patient variables in, 154–156
  prediction in, 156–159, *157, 158*
Dead space, physiologic, ventilation status and, 144
Decision making
  computers and, 150–151
  data processing and, 153–156
Dehydration, nonrebreathing systems and, 17–18
Delivery system. *See also* specific systems.
  Alabama. *See* Alabama Automated Closed-Circuit Anesthesia System.
  Arizona. *See* Arizona system.
  Boston. *See* Boston system.
  classification of, 11–12, 12t
  new. *See also* Future of anesthesia.
    design of
      breathing circuit in, 94
      function in, 90–91
      gas proportionating systems in, 91–93
    microprocessor control in, 95–96
    need for, 4–7
    requirements in, 91, *92*
    sensors in, 94–95
    ventilators in, 96–97
    volatile anesthetic delivery systems in, 93–94
    economic considerations in, 5–6
    medicolegal considerations in, 5
    need for, 3–7
    safety and, 6–7
  Utah. *See* Utah system.
Denitrogenation, rebreathing system and, 28
Depth of anesthesia, gas concentration monitoring and, 140–141, 141t
Design of systems. *See* Delivery systems, new, design of.
Dinamap automatic blood pressure recording device, 69
Disconnection, alarm for, 70
Display of data, centralized, 152
Dot Spectral Array system, 198

EFFICIENCY, nonrebreathing system, 14–15
Electrocardiograph
  data processing and, 154–155, *154*
  endotracheal tubes and, 195–196
  esophageal multiprobe and, 195
Electroencephalograph, Arizona system and, 196–198
Electromyography
  Arizona system and, 198
  muscle relaxation and, computers in, 55
Electronic control, equipment design and, 241
Enflurane
  monitoring of, 138, 140
  standard dosages of, 29t, 30t
Engineering, human
  computers and, 159
  problems on, 159
  standards of, 68–69
Engstrom EMMA, 181
Equipment selection. *See* Future of anesthesia, equipment selection and.
Exhalation, measurement of, rebreathing systems and, 21–22

FEEDBACK
    closed loop system and, 128
    control and, Utah system and, 221–222, 223, 228–229, *229*
    flowmeter, 201
Fick principle, 20, 144
Filter, charcoal, rebreathing systems and, 26–28, *26, 27,* 31
Fittings, standards for
    material, 64–65
    size, 61–64
Flow controllers, 104–105
Flow rate. *See also* Flowmeter.
    Arizona system and, 198–200
    Boston system and, 211
    conservation of mass and, 100–101
    delivery system classification by, 11–12, 12t,
    mass balance equation and, 100–101
    mathematical formulations of, 146–147
    ranges of, 99
    Utah system and, 228
Flowmeter. *See also* Flow rate.
    design of, problems in, 92–93
    ideal, 101
    linear resistance laminar, 104, 194, 201
    pitot tube, 104, 195
    pneumotachometer and, disposable, 195
    problems of, 102–103
    structure of, 103–104
    thermal, 104
    venturi, 104
Fluerics, definition of, 8
Fluid requirements, oxygen consumption and, *20,* 21
Fluidics
    definition of, 7–8
    system design and, 90, 93
Fluorocarbons, ozone depletion and, 16–17
Funnel, computer as, 152–153
Future of anesthesia. *See also* Delivery systems, new.
    equipment selection and
        convenience in, 240
        glamor in, 240
        manufacturer's hyperbole in, 241–242
        obsolescence in, 239–240, 242–243

safety in, 239
specification development in, 240–241
planning for, 237

GAS. *See also* specific gases.
    concentration of
        conservation of mass and, 141, 146
        Fick principle and, 144
        mass balance and, 142, *143,* 147–148
        mathematical formulations of, 146–148
    monitoring of
        depth of anesthesia and, 140–141, 141t
        physiologic variables and, 141–144, *142,* 142t
        reasons for, 137–138, 138t
        targets of, 138
    partial rebreathing system and, 18
    delivery of. *See also* Delivery system.
        flow controllers and, 104–105
        flowmeters and. *See* Flowmeters.
        problems of, 102–103
        safety features and, 103
        techniques of
            current, 102–103
            future, 103–106
        ventilator and, integration of, 171–172
    mixing of
        definition of, 100
        equipment for, 105–106
    proportionating of
        Arizona, 198–201, *199, 200*
        definition of, 100
        design of, problems in, 91–93
        equipment for, 105–106
    sensors of. *See* Sensors, gas.
Gas waste. *See* Waste gases.
Greenhouse effect
    halothane and, 117–118
    nitrous oxide and, 117

HALOTHANE
    concentrations of
        charcoal filtration and, *27*
        monitoring of, 138, 140
        drug metabolism and, increased, 112

Halothane—*continued*
  efficiency and, nonrebreathing system and, 14
  greenhouse effect and, 117–118
  standard dosages of, 29t, 30t
  uptake of, square root of time model for, *33*, 34–36, *34*
  vigilance monitoring of, 140
Heat loss, rebreathing systems and, 17–18
Human engineering
  computers and, 159
  problems of, 159
  standards of, 68–69
Human error, incidence of, 6
Hydrogen, rebreathing systems and, 25
Hyperthermia, malignant, oxygen consumption and, 21
Hyperthyroidism, acute, oxygen consumption and, 21

INFORMATION processing, decision making and, 155–156. *See also* Data processing.
Isoflurane
  concentrations of, monitoring of, 138
  standard dosages of, 29t, 30t
  vigilance monitoring of, 140

JET edge oscillator, Arizona system and, 188–191, *189, 190*

LABELS
  ampule, standards for, 75–76
  syringe, colors of, 73–75, 74t
Leakage
  rebreathing system and, 25
  waste gases and, 113–114
Leasing of equipment, 242–243
Litigation, new delivery systems and, 5
Luer Taper fittings, standards and, 65
Lung-thorax compliance, monitoring of, 170, 171

MASK adapter
  multiple, 59–61, *60*
  pediatric, 63–64, *63*
Methane, rebreathing systems and, 25
Microelectronics, anesthesia and, 8
Microprocessor. *See* Computers.
Modeling, dynamic system and, 156–159, *157, 158*

Modularity, equipment design and, 241
Monitoring. *See also* Sensors.
  carbon dioxide. *See* Carbon dioxide.
  cerebral function, 197
  closed loop control systems and, 129, 134
  electrocardiographic, data processing and, 154–155, *154*
  gas concentration. *See* Gas, concentration of, monitoring of.
  oxygen. *See* Oxygen.
  pressure, 168–169, 170
  rebreathing systems and. *See* Rebreathing systems, monitoring in.
  vigilance
    elements of, 139, 139t
    need for, 139–140
Muscle relaxants, monitoring of, computers in, 55

NARCOTIC-relaxant-nitrous oxide-oxygen anesthetic, rebreathing system and, 28, 28t
Needle valves, problems of, 102
Neuromuscular block, control systems and, 134
Nitrogen concentration
  monitoring of, 24–25
  rebreathing systems and, 24–25, 28
Nitrous oxide
  concentration of
    Arizona system and, 198–199
    depth of anesthesia and, 140, 141t
    monitoring of, 138, 139t, 140
  efficiency and, nonrebreathing system and, 14–15
  exposure levels of, operating room, 113
  greenhouse effect and, 117
  recycling of, 114, 119, 121
  scavenging systems and, 114
  uptake of, Utah system and, 230
  ventilation and, high-frequency, 173
  waste, atmosphere and, 115–118, *116*
Nonrebreathing system, total. *See also* Rebreathing system, partial.
  cost and, 15–16, 15t
  dehydration and, 17–18
  federal regulations and, 17
  gas waste and, 15
  operating room ventilation and, 16
  ozone depletion and, 16–17

OBSOLESCENCE, equipment selection and, 239–240, 242–243
Open system. *See* Nonrebreathing system.
Oxygen
  concentration of
    Arizona system and, 199–200
    Boston system and, 213–214
    closed loop control systems and, 131
    computers and, 54
    depth of anesthesia and, 140, 141t
    monitoring of, 138, 139–140, 139t, 170, 180–182, *182*, 231
    Utah system and, 228–229, 231
  consumption of
    acute hyperthyroidism and, 21
    Fick principle and, 20
    malignant hyperthermia and, 21
    measurement of, 19–21, *20*
    pain and, 230
    Utah system and, 222–224, *225*, 229–230
    weight and, 19, *20*
  delivery of, theory of, 177–178
  efficiency and, nonrebreathing system and, 14–15
  mass flow rates of, 142
  monitoring of
    Alabama system and, 180–182, *182*
    rebreathing systems and, 23–24, 28, 28t
    standards of, 68
    vigilance, 139–140, 139t
    Utah system and, 231
  safety features and, 103
Oxygen analyzer
  alarms and, 69
  rebreathing systems and, 23–24, 28, 28t
Ozone destruction
  halogenated agents and, 118
  nitrous oxide and, 115–116, *116*
  nonrebreathing systems and, 16–17

PITOT tube, 104, 195
Pneumatics, definition of, 8
Pneumotachometer, disposable, 195
Pollution, anesthesia
    environment and, 16–17
    operating room and, 16

Pop-off valve
  nonrebreathing system and, 14
  partial rebreathing system and, 12, 18
Prediction
  computers and, 150–151
  dynamic system and, 156–159, *157, 158*
Proportional-integral-derivative scheme, feedback controller and, 223, *224*
Psychomotor effects, waste gases and, 112
Pulmonary dynamics, quantitative, 21–23, *22*
Purchase of equipment. *See* Future of anesthesia, equipment selection and.

REBREATHING system. *See also* specific systems.
  balanced anesthesia and, 28, 28t
  charcoal shunt and, 26–28, *26, 27,* 31
  definition of, 12, 12t, *13*
  dual-flow ranges and, 93
  exhalation in, measurement of, 21–22
  monitoring in
    carbon dioxide, *20*, 21
    fluid requirements, *20*, 21
    oxygen consumption, 19–21, *20*
    variables of, 19
  partial
    definition of, 12, 12t, *13*
    disadvantages of, 18
    gas concentration and, 18
    waste gases and, operating room and, 113
  prime dose calculation in, 36
  problems of
    agent concentration and, 24
    anesthesia emergence and, 26–28, *26, 27*
    hypoxia and, 23–24
    mechanical, 25
    medicolegal, 25–26
    nitrogen concentration and, 24–25
    volatile agents and, 25, 26–28, *26*
    quantitative pulmonary dynamics and, 21–23, *22*
    tidal volumes and, 21–23, *22*

INDEX 251

Rebreathing system—*continued*
 total
  advantages of, 14–15
  definition of, 12, 12t, *13*
  disadvantages of, heat loss and, 17–18
  unit dose calculation in, 35–36
  uptake predictions in
   square root of time model and, 32–36, *34,* 35t
   Züntz equation and, 31–32, 33
Redundancy, equipment design and, 241
Rental of equipment, 242–243
Requirements, general, system design and, 91, *92*
Rotameter
 design of, 91–93
 inaccuracies of, 194
 problems of, 91–93, 102, 194
 structure of, 103–104
 vaporizers and, 106
Rowland-Molina hypothesis, 16–17

SAFETY
 Boston system and, 213
 equipment selection and, 239
 gas delivery and, 103
Scavenging systems, waste gases and, 113–114, 119
Sensors. *See also* Monitoring.
 Arizona system. *See* Arizona system, sensors of.
 design of, 94–95
 electrolyte, 195
 flow. *See* Flowmeters.
 gas. *See also* Flowmeters.
  design of, 94–95
  electromechanical, 191–194, *193*
  flueric oscillator, 188–191, *189, 190*
  functions of, 94–95
  linear resistor-orifice, 191, *192*
 oxygen
  Boston system and, 213–214
  Utah system and, 223
 pH, 195
 physiologic
  blood pressure and, 196, 197
  central nervous system monitoring and, 196–198
  endotracheal multiprobes and, 195–196
  esophageal multiprobes and, 195–196
 ion specific field effect transistors and, 195
Siemens Servoventilator, Utah system and, 226–227
Specifications, development of, 240–241. *See also* specific systems.
Spirometer ventilator, rebreathing system and, 21–23, *22*
Square root of time model, uptake predictions and, 32–36, *34,* 35t
Standards
 alarm, 69–71, 70t
 American National Committee Z79 on, 61–64, 79–84
 American Society of Anesthetists Committee on, 61–64
 breathing circuit layout, 65–67
 color
  syringe labels and, 73–75, 74t
  volatile anesthetic containers and, 72–73, 72t
 Compressed Gas Association and, 66
 disconnections and, 61–65, 68
 FDA Bureau of Medical Devices on, 71–77, 72t, 74t
 fittings and, 61–65, 68
 future, 68–69
 history of, 63–64
 human engineering and, 68–69
 International Standards Organization and, 85–86
 mask adapter and
  multiple, 59–61, *60*
  pediatric, 63–64, *63*
 oxygen monitor, 68
 performance
  breathing system, 67–68
  FDA and, 71–72
 pharmaceuticals and, 75–77
 tubing compliance and, 67–68
 ventilators and, 67
Stress, anesthetist, 7
Syringe, drugs in, emergencies and, 76–77
Syringe pump, Arizona system and, 201

TEK type vaporizer, rebreathing system and, 28–30, 29t, 30t
Transistors, ion specific field effect, 195

UPTAKE predictions
  square root of time model for, 32–36, *34,* 35t
  Züntz equation for, 31–32, *33*
Utah system
  carbon dioxide absorber and, 223
  clinical application of, 229–230
  current configuration of, 228–229, *229*
  development of, 222–228, *223, 224, 225, 226, 227*
  error signal in, 223–224
  feedback in
    control and, 221–222, 223, 228–229, *229*
    nitrous oxide and, 225, *225*
    ventilation and, 226–227, *226*
  flow rate in, 228
  future of, 230–231
  gas analyzer in, 228
  nitrous oxide uptake in, 230
  oxygen concentration in, 228–229
  oxygen consumption and, 222–224, *225,* 229–230
  vapor concentration and, 227–228, *227*
  xenon anesthesia and, 226

VALVES
  binary, 105
  flueric vortex, 105
  needle, 102, 104
  time-controlled, 105
Vapor concentration, Utah system and, 227–228, *227*
Vapor delivery
  energy and, 106–107
  ideal, 101–102
  problems of, 106
  techniques of
    current, 106
    future, 107
Vaporizer, Tek type, 29–30, 29t, 30t
Variables
  availability of, computers and, 151–152
  physiologic, gas concentration monitoring and, 141–144, *142,* 142t
  respiratory, mathematical formulations of, 148
Ventilation. *See also* Ventilators.
  Alabama system and, 181
  assessment of, 144
  high-frequency, 172–173

  jet, 172–173, 204
  monitoring of, computers and, 54
  operating room
    nonrebreathing system and, 16–17
    waste gases and, 113–114
  oscillation, high-frequency, 172–173, 204
  positive pressure, high-frequency, 172
  rate of, theory of, 178–179
  Utah system and, 226–227, *226,* 229
Ventilators. *See also* Ventilation.
  accessory nature of, anesthesia machine and, 170–171
  Air Shields Ventimeter, 179–181
  anesthesia machine and, integration of, 171–172
  Arizona system, 202–204, 202t, *203*
  Boston system, 213–214
  design of, future, 96–97
  high-frequency, 203–204
  ideal
    alarms and, 168–169
    bellows and, 167, 168–169
    body size and, 166–167
    compactness and, 167–168
    computers and, 168
    cost and, 169
    energy efficiency and, 169
    feedback control and, 170
    intensive care unit and, 167
    modes and, 167
    monitors and, 168–169, 170
    positive end expiratory pressure and, 167
    pressure monitors and, 168–169, 170
    reliability and, 165–166
    safety and, 168–169
    servo control and, 170
    versatility and, 166–167
  pediatric, 203, *203*
  spirometer, 21–23, *22*
  standards for, 67
  time-cycled, 166
  volume-cycled, 166
Ventimeter ventilator, 21, *22*
Venturi meter, 104
Volatile agent
  concentration of
    computers and, 55
    monitoring of, 138, 139t, 140

INDEX 253

Volatile agent—*continued*
  containers for, colors of, 72–73, 72t
  delivery of
    Alabama system and, 181
    analyzer of, 181
    Arizona system and, 201
    Boston system and, 211–212
    design of, 93–94
    theory of, 178
    vaporization and, 106
  dosages of, standard, 29t, 30t
  greenhouse effect and, 117–118
  high-frequency ventilation and, 173
  monitoring of, electromechanical, 191–194, *193,* 204
  rebreathing systems and, 25, 26–31, *26,* 29t, 30t
  recovery of, 201–202
  removal of, waste gas recycling and, 119, 222

WASTE gases
  atmosphere and, effects on, 115–118, *116*
  closed circuits and, 111
  effects of, operating room and, 112
  environments and, 110, *111*
  exposure levels of, recommended, 113
  high-flow techniques and, 5–6
  nitrous oxide, atmosphere and, 115–117, *116*
  nonrebreathing systems and, 15–16
  operating room and
    controversy of, 112
    effects in, 112
    partial rebreathing systems and, 113
  ozone destruction and, 115–116, *116*
  reasons for, 111–112
  rebreathing systems and, 15t, 18
  recovery of
    cost-benefit analysis of, 121–122
    problems of, 121
    system for, 118–121, *120*
  removal of, operating room and, 113–114
  scavenging systems and, 113–114, 119
  sources of, 113
  volatile, removal of, 119, 122

XENON anesthesia, Utah system and, 226

ZÜNTZ equation, uptake prediction and, 31–32, 33